WHAT YOU MUST KNOW ABOUT
DRY EYE

HOW TO PREVENT, STOP, OR REVERSE DRY EYE DISEASE

JEFFREY ANSHEL, OD

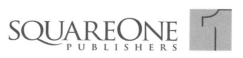

SQUAREONE
PUBLISHERS

The information and advice contained in this book are based upon the research and the personal and professional experiences of the author. They are not intended as a substitute for consulting with a healthcare professional. The publisher and author are not responsible for any adverse effects or consequences resulting from the use of any of the suggestions, preparations, or procedures discussed in this book. All matters pertaining to your physical health should be supervised by a healthcare professional. It is a sign of wisdom, not cowardice, to seek a second or third opinion. \

COVER DESIGNER: Jeannie Rosado
IN-HOUSE EDITOR: Michael Weatherhead
TYPESETTER: Gary A. Rosenberg

Square One Publishers
115 Herricks Road
Garden City Park, NY 11040
(516) 535-2010 * (877) 900-BOOK

Library of Congress Cataloging-in-Publication Data
Names: Anshel, Jeffrey, author.
Title: What you must know about dry eye : how to prevent, stop, or reverse
  dry eye disease / Jeffrey Anshel, OD.
Description: Garden City Park, NY : Square One Publishers, [2019] | Includes
  bibliographical references and index.
Identifiers: LCCN 2019018125 (print) | LCCN 2019021630 (ebook) | ISBN
  9780757054792 (e-book) | ISBN 9780757004797 (pbk.)
Subjects: LCSH: Dry eye syndromes.
Classification: LCC RE216.D78 (ebook) | LCC RE216.D78 A57 2019 (print) | DDC
  617.7—dc23
LC record available at https://lccn.loc.gov/2019018125

Figure 4.1. Ocular Surface Disease Index reprinted courtesy of Allergan plc.

Figure 4.2. Dry Eye Questionnaire 5 reprinted courtesy of Indiana University.

Figure 4.3. Standardized Patient Evaluation of Eye Dryness reprinted courtesy of TearScience, Inc.

Printed in the United States of America

10   9   8   7   6   5   4   3   2   1

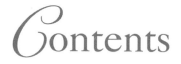

Contents

This book is dedicated to my son, Casey Heaton,
who has always supported my role in his life,
and who continues to show me how to live
my life to its fullest potential.

Acknowledgments

First and foremost, I would like to acknowledge the support of my mentor, Ellen Troyer, MT, MA, who has dedicated her professional career to addressing dry eye disease through nutrition, and who is always willing to share her knowledge and passion with all eyecare professionals and their patients.

I would also like to acknowledge my partner, Ginnie Mathews, who has supported my work wholeheartedly and unconditionally with her love and caring.

Introduction

Despite the fact that we count on our eyes for so much in life, most people take the health of these important organs for granted until vision problems arise. Whether you are currently experiencing issues with your eyes and have questions, or you simply want to preserve your eyesight for years to come, you will find this book contains valuable information to meet your needs.

It is only in the past several decades that a significant, international research effort has been directed towards understanding the composition and regulation of the tear film that covers the front of the eye. This effort recognizes that the tear film plays a critical role in maintaining the integrity of the cornea and conjunctiva, protecting against undesirable microbes, and preserving visual clarity. In addition, research has been stimulated by the knowledge that alterations to or deficiencies in the tear film, which occur in innumerable individuals throughout the world, may lead to eye dryness, ulcer formation in the cornea, an increased incidence of infectious disease, and potentially pronounced visual disabilities and blindness.

The goal of this book is to give you a voice in your interactions with your eyecare professional so that your dry eye condition can be resolved quickly and completely. Shared decision-making is a key component of patient-centered healthcare, in which doctors and patients work together to make decisions and select tests and treatments based on science that balances risks and expected outcomes with patient preferences and values. Shared decision-making helps doctors and patients agree on a healthcare plan. If you participate in the decision-making and understand what you need to do, you are more likely to follow through with your therapy and achieve a successful outcome. Often, there is more than one reasonable option, or no single option that has a clear advantage.

This book takes a close look at dry eye disease, from the basics of this condition to how you can take advantage of personalized medical treatments and lifestyle modifications to resolve it. Part One begins by providing the reader with some basic information on the eyeball, including a detailed breakdown of the anatomy of the eye, a description of how the eye sees, and an explanation of the importance of the tear film to eye health. It then defines dry eye and outlines its effects on vision and eye health. Finally, it lists the many causes of dry eye and the ways in which a doctor can test for this condition.

Part Two deals with the treatment of dry eye, focusing first on the numerous medical therapies available, such as artificial tears, anti-evaporatives, and prescription drugs. From there, it takes a nutritional approach to dry eye therapy. It describes how oxidative stress and inflammation are associated with dry eye disease, and then details the nutrients that have proven effective in tempering these issues. Finally, it provides a list of foods that contain significant amounts of these nutrients and suggests supplements that can fill in any gaps in your diet.

Once you have a firm grasp on the basis of your dry eye condition and how you can alleviate it, you will be able to bring all the tools at your disposal together and use them to move past this debilitating problem and the daily impairment it causes.

PART ONE

Dry Eye Basics

In order to know how the condition of dry eye can affect your eyes and visual system, it's important to become familiar with the basic anatomy of the eye. The first part of this book begins by describing the structure of the eye, how light enters this organ, the path light travels once it enters the eye, and how images are formed in the brain. It then explains how dry eye is currently defined, the different types of dry eye, and the effects this condition can have on your eyesight and eye health. Finally, it details the most common causes of dry eye and provides helpful information on how doctors test for dry eye, allowing you to feel confident in having a dialogue with your eyecare provider in regard to your possible dry eye condition and what your next steps should be if you have it.

1

$\mathcal{E}$yeball Basics

Like most people with eye conditions, you probably never thought about the health of your eyes until a problem arose. More than likely, you've been concerned only with how clearly you can see when driving or reading. If you are affected by dry eye and have seen your doctor about it, you may have found it difficult to understand the clinical explanation of this condition. When trying to determine the contributing factors of dry eye, doctors consider not only the tear film of each eye but also other anatomical features. If you don't know much about the structure of your eyes and lack a basic idea of how your eyes work, you won't be able to comprehend fully what is happening to them. This chapter aims to give you a basic sense of the different structures of the eye and how they relate to each other. Hopefully you can use this information to present your eye doctor with a more accurate description of any eye health or vision issue you may be experiencing.

THE ANATOMY OF THE EYE

Although it is only about an inch in diameter and three inches in circumference, the eye is one of the most complex organs of the human body. This slightly asymmetrical globe has many parts that work together to provide you with your sense of sight. (See Figure 1.1. "The Anatomy of the Eye" on page 6.)

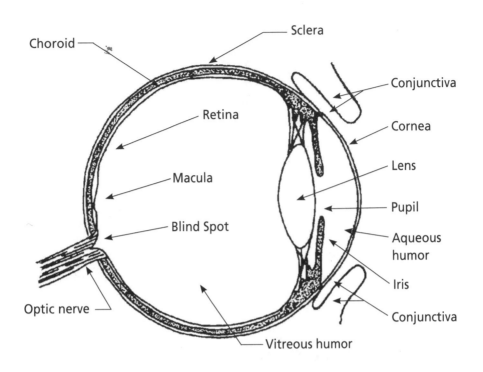

Choroid

Sclera

Conjunctiva

Retina

Cornea

Macula

Lens

Blind Spot

Pupil

Aqueous humor

Iris

Optic nerve

Conjunctiva

Vitreous humor

Figure 1.1. The Anatomy of the Eye.

SCLERA

The *sclera* is the dense white outer covering of the eye that is otherwise known as the white of the eye. The main purpose of this vital part of the eye is to provide support and protection for the inner eye structures and to attach the eye to the six muscles that control its movement up and down and from side to side.

The cells that make up the sclera are white in color, but some blood vessels do pass through the sclera towards other tissues. When these vessels become swollen or dilated, the eyes may appear bloodshot, which refers to a redness of the eyes. More often, though, a reddish looking eye is the result of irritation to the *conjunctiva,* which is the thin, normally transparent membrane that covers the sclera and lines the inside of the eyelids.

CHOROID

Located just inside the sclera, covering the same area as the sclera, is the *choroid*. The middle layer of the eye wall, the choroid is sandwiched between the sclera and the very thin light-sensitive inner layer known as the retina. The choroid is made up of blood vessels that deliver oxygen and nutrients to the retina. It also provides oxygen and nutrients to other structures found inside the eye.

CORNEA

The *cornea* is the transparent dome-shaped structure that covers the front of the eye. Together with the sclera, it makes up the outer surface of the eyeball and supports the eye's internal structures. The cornea also acts as the eye's outermost lens, functioning as a window that helps control the entry of light into the eye. When light hits the cornea, the cornea refracts (bends) the light through the lens as it makes its way back to the retina. In fact, the cornea provides up to 75 percent of the eye's focusing power.

Unlike the vast majority of the structures in the body, the cornea does not contain any blood vessels. Instead, it receives nourishment from the tear film that covers it and from the aqueous humor, which is directly behind it.

AQUEOUS HUMOR

The *aqueous humor* is a clear fluid that fills the small chamber between the cornea, which is in front of it, and the iris, which is behind it. The aqueous humor holds much of the nutrition that supports the tissues in this area, which include the lens of the eye. The aqueous humor flows into and out of the eye on a regular basis. When this flow is not properly controlled, potentially damaging eye pressure conditions such as *glaucoma*, which refers to abnormally high eye pressure, can result.

IRIS AND PUPIL

The *iris* is the colored portion of the eye found in front of the lens. (See the following discussion on the lens.) This ring-shaped structure regulates the amount of light that enters the eye through the *pupil*, the round opening in the center of the iris. When you look directly at someone's eye, the pupil looks like a black spot in the middle of the colored iris. The iris contains muscles that allow the pupil to get bigger (to open up or dilate) when there is relatively little light, or to get smaller (close up or constrict) when the light is bright.

LENS

Situated behind the iris, the *lens,* also called the *crystalline lens,* is a transparent structure made of flexible tissue. It is biconvex in shape, meaning that it is thicker in the middle and thinner on the edges. The lens's elasticity allows it to change shape and focus on objects that are different distances from the eye. When the lens is stretched and thin, it can focus on distant objects. When it becomes thicker and more rounded, it increases in power and can focus on objects that are closer. The ciliary muscles attached to the lens facilitate these shape changes. The lens is the second part of the eye that works to focus images on the retina, the first being the cornea.

A healthy lens is clear. When it has developed what is known as a *cataract,* or a clouding of the lens, vision is affected.

VITREOUS HUMOR

The *vitreous humor* is a clear gel-like substance that fills the large central chamber of the eye between the lens and the retina. Because the gel is firm, it helps maintain the spherical shape of the eye and supports the retina. Because it is clear, light can easily pass through it. Unlike the aqueous humor, which flows into and out of the eye, the vitreous humor is a stagnant (unmoving) fluid. If a substance enters this gel, it remains suspended there. These suspended substances are collectively referred to as *floaters*. During the prenatal stage of development, blood vessels grow through the vitreous humor to feed the developing front of the eye. Just prior to birth, these blood vessels dissolve—mostly. Those cells that do not dissolve remain suspended in the middle of the vitreous.

Throughout most of your life, you typically do not notice these small cells, but as you age, the vitreous humor softens into a fluid gel, and these cells begin to "float" around. When they move near the retina or macula and you look at a bright light, the floaters can cast shadows on the retina, appearing as black spots or threadlike fibers. New floaters can also form when *protein* fibers from the vitreous gel clump together. It is normal to see some floaters as you age, but if you suddenly begin seeing large numbers of them, it is important to contact your doctor, as this can be a sign of a detached retina or another retinal disease.

RETINA AND MACULA

The *retina* is a thin layer of tissue that lines the back of the eye. The purpose of this structure is to receive the light that is focused by the lens, convert it into neural signals, and send the signal to the brain for interpretation. Human beings have what is sometimes called a "camera-type eye." The cornea and lens focus light onto the light-sensitive retina just as a camera lens focuses light onto film.

The central part of the retina, called the *macula*, offers sharp, detailed vision—the type of vision needed to thread a needle or read a book. Visual acuity is highest in the *fovea*, a small dimple found in the middle of the macula. We refer to the fovea and the macula as the *macular region*. When we discuss macular degeneration, we refer to this region.

The retina is composed of several layers of cells, and one layer is embedded with specialized cells known as *rods* and *cones*. Called *photoreceptors* because they respond to light, each of these cell types has a particular function. The long, slender cells known as rods are responsible for vision in low levels of light, and therefore are essential to night vision. Cones, on the other hand, are active in higher levels of light and respond to colors, and therefore are essential to daytime vision. Our sharpest vision comes from the cones, which work under most light conditions and provide detail.

Rods and cones are not evenly distributed throughout the retina. Cones are found in greatest concentration in the area of the macula, and rods are found in the outer edges of the retina. This is why the most important detailed images are formed at the macula, while the rest of the retina provides peripheral vision—the vision at the edge of the visual field. When cones and rods receive information provided by light, they convert this information into electrical signals, which are then transmitted to the brain via the optic nerve.

OPTIC NERVE

Located in the back of the eye, just off the center of the retina, the *optic nerve* uses electrical impulses to transfer the visual information received by the retina to the vision centers of the brain. The retina, which is described in detail in the previous section, contains *ganglion cells*, which are specialized nerve cells that receive signals from the rod and cone photoreceptors. The optic nerve is composed of the thread-like fibers of the ganglion cells, with each optic nerve—one from each eye—containing about one million nerve fibers. The two optic nerves meet in the brain, where the electrical impulses are converted into images.

HOW THE EYE SEES

Vision begins when light passes through the cornea, which starts the focusing process by bending the light so that it can enter the eye. The light then moves through the aqueous humor, through the pupil, through the lens, where the image is further focused, and then through the vitreous humor. Finally, the image is focused onto the retina (most acutely onto the macular area), where the light stimulates the rod and cone cells. The rods and cones convert the light into electrical signals, which are sent to the visual cortex of the brain via the optic nerve. The brain then reconciles the two slightly different images it receives—one from each eye—and creates a single image. Thus, your vision is really the result of two processes: (1) the eye receiving light, and (2) the brain interpreting the signals from the eye.

THE IMPORTANCE OF THE TEAR FILM

While the cornea is considered the first anatomical structure of the eye that light passes through as it makes its way into the eye, technically the first surface that light meets is the *tear film*, or *precorneal film*, which floats in front of the cornea. The integrity of the tear film is important in maintaining the optical quality of the image the eye receives. The aqueous fluid inside the anterior chamber of the eye and the tear film on the outside of the cornea both contribute to the integrity and moisture of the cornea.

There are several types of tears that are produced by *lacrimal glands* in several places around the eye. The first type is called *basal tears*, which are produced by glands in the conjunctiva. They lubricate the eye and keep it clear of dust and debris. The second type is known as *reflex tears*, which are produced and secreted in response to the presence of an irritant such a foreign body or irritant fumes. The third type is called *psychic tears*, which occur in response to strong emotions, such as sadness, extreme stress, or even happiness.

Despite the fact that the tear film is extremely thin—about 3 microns (3 millionths of a meter) across (a human hair is about 75 microns)—it comprises three general layers: the *mucin layer*, the *aqueous layer*, and the *lipid layer*. These layers are not separated by any particular structure, so they are somewhat blended together, with the density of the proteins in the tears defining the different layers.

Mucin Layer

The mucin layer is the innermost layer of the tear film, closest to the cornea. Produced predominantly by goblet cells in the conjunctiva, *mucins* are proteins that form a gel-like coating of mucus over the cornea. This layer of mucus allows the watery layer above it to wet the surface of the cornea evenly, aiding in the retention of moisture. In addition to assisting in the lubrication of the cornea, the mucin layer also acts as a protective barrier against bacteria and viruses.

Aqueous Layer

Produced by the lacrimal glands, the aqueous layer is the thickest portion of the tear film. As its name suggests, it is the watery component of the tear film. It hydrates the cornea, flushes out particles, and helps prevent infection. It also contains many of the nutrients that support the health of the cornea.

Lipid Layer

The lipid layer is the outermost portion of the tear film. It is produced by the *meibomian glands*, which are located within the structure of the eyelids. These glands produce the oils that make up the lipid layer, which are squeezed out of these glands and spread over the eye with each blink. This oil-based component coats the aqueous layer, providing a seal for the tear film, which reduces evaporation of the tear layers below and limits any spillage of tears onto the cheeks.

CONCLUSION

Now that you are familiar with the anatomical structure of the eye and how it functions to provide you with your sense of sight, you are better equipped to understand eye problems and how they can impact your eyesight and lifestyle. Having learned about the tear film, you may already have some ideas about what dry eye is and what causes this condition. The following chapter will define this troubling disorder and provide information regarding its development and effects.

2

*W*hat Is Dry Eye?

Known by a variety of names, including *dry eye syndrome, dry eye disease, ocular surface disease,* and just plain *dry eye,* this common ocular disorder is one of the main reasons for visits to the eye doctor. Unfortunately, as dry eye is not necessarily a sight-threatening condition, many health and eyecare professionals do not think it deserves much thought. If you are affected by dry eye, however, you know how frustrating it is and how damaging it can be to your life. The fact is that dry eye can make even the simplest task difficult to accomplish.

Dry eye may result from disruption of the production of any tear film component, alteration of the distribution of tears, or disturbance of the tear film layers. Although each form of dry eye may exist in isolation, frequently there is a mixed presentation depending upon the underlying disease process and its duration.

While this condition might seem straightforward, the definition of dry eye has been many years in the making. In the 1970s, once doctors began to recognize a similar series of physical symptoms in their patients, they started to refer to them collectively as *dry eye syndrome* (DES), also called *keratoconjunctivitis sicca* (KCS). In general, it was considered a disorder of the tear film caused by diminished tear production or excessive tear evaporation. Many factors became associated with the possible onset of dry eye. As the number of people affected by this problem grew, so did the number of factors thought to contribute to dry eye. This increase in awareness led to the

American Optometric Association to define dry eye as "any condition that reduces the production, alters the composition, or impedes the distribution of the pre-ocular tear film may cause a noticeable degradation of vision and irritation to the structures of the front surface of the eye."

In 2006, a group of international professional researchers known as the Delphi Panel convened to develop treatment recommendations for dry eye patients. This panel proposed a new term for the condition: *dysfunctional tear syndrome* (DTS). The main outcome of this convention was treatment recommendations for different types and severity levels of dry eye disease, which were based primarily on patient symptoms and signs.

In 2007, Tear Film and Ocular Surface Society (TFOS) created a "Dry Eye Workshop" (DEWS) made up of international eyecare professionals involved in the study of dry eye. These professionals were charged with developing a new definition of the condition. The workshop termed the problem *dry eye disease* (DED) and defined it as "a multifactorial disease of the tears and ocular surface that results in symptoms of discomfort, visual disturbance, and tear film instability with potential damage to the ocular surface. It is accompanied by increased osmolarity [salt concentration] of the tear film and inflammation of the ocular surface."

In 2017, TFOS reassembled its Dry Eye Workshop. Known as DEWS II, this workshop published an updated version of the original DEWS report. As part of this update, the group formulated a new definition of dry eye disease, which states, "Dry eye disease is a multifactorial disease of the ocular surface characterized by a loss of homeostasis (physiological balance) of the tear film, and accompanied by ocular symptoms, in which tear film instability and hyperosmolarity, ocular surface inflammation and damage, and neurosensory abnormalities play etiological roles." This definition expands upon the 2007 description to include more known causes and ramifications of the disease. Currently, the term *ocular surface disease* (OSD) has come to be used interchangeably with the term dry eye disease by eyecare professionals.

Clearly, whether it is called a syndrome, disease, disorder, or condition, dry eye is a problem whose definition is still a work in progress. As the science of tear chemistry continues to develop, it is likely that more details of dry eye will become known and lead to better treatment options or, hopefully, prevention of this condition.

TYPES OF DRY EYE

There are two general types of dry eye. The first is known as *aqueous tear-deficient dry eye* and is associated with dysfunction in your tear glands. This dysfunction makes your tear glands unable to produce a sufficient amount of tears. The second is known as *evaporative dry eye*. Unlike tear-deficient dry eye, evaporative dry eye is not associated with a problem in tear production. Instead, it refers to when your tears evaporate too quickly from the surface of your eye. In spite of their differences, both types of dry eye will alter the tear film of the eye and therefore affect your vision.

Aqueous Tear-Deficient Dry Eye

Several glands located in and around your eye produce tears. As discussed in Chapter 1, there are lacrimal glands within the conjunctiva (transparent covering over the white of the eye) that produce basal tears, which maintain normal moisture of the surface of your eye and protect it from dust and debris. In addition, lacrimal glands, or tear glands, located above your eye and within the bone behind your eyebrow, are responsible for the flush of tears needed to rid your eye of foreign particles or irritant fumes.

These glands are categorized as *exocrine glands* because they produce and secrete substances onto *epithelial cells*, which make up the tissues that line the outer surfaces of organs and blood vessels, by way of ducts. If they do not produce enough tears for any reason, you will likely be affected by aqueous tear-deficient dry eye.

Evaporative Dry Eye

Every time you blink, you spread a new layer of much-needed tears onto the front of each of your corneas. This blinking action serves to clean the front surface of the eye as well as to refresh the tear film. As explained in Chapter 1, the tear film is made up of three layers. The outermost layer, known as the lipid layer, is created by secretions of the meibomian glands, which produce the oils that form this front layer of the tear film. If this lipid layer is not uniform, or if it is not strong enough to maintain its structural integrity, the tears in the aqueous layer beneath it will evaporate far too quickly, leading to evaporative dry eye.

Evaporative dry eye can be categorized by cause. These distinctions include:

Mucin-Deficient Dry Eye

This category of evaporative dry eye disease is caused by a decrease in the production of mucus due to a reduction in the number of conjunctival cells. The conjunctival cells may experience a reduction in connection with any health condition that is damaging to the conjunctiva.

Lipid-Abnormality Dry Eye

This category of evaporative dry eye is typically associated with eyelid disorders brought about by inflammation, trauma, or scarring after eyelid surgery. It is most often caused by chronic inflammation of glands in and around the eyelids.

Surfacing Abnormalities

This distinction refers to any structural defect of the lid that can interfere with tear film distribution. Such a defect may lead to an impairment of normal blinking action (e.g., incomplete or infrequent blinking), which can result in excessive tear evaporation, or prevent efficient resurfacing of the tear layer, as can be the case with drooping eyelids or loss of eyelashes.

Irregular Corneal Surface

Evaporative dry eye can also be caused by an irregular corneal surface, which may prevent mucin from adhering to the cornea. An irregular corneal surface may arise from a number of conditions, including corneal scarring, corneal erosion, chemical burns, and contact lens complications.

The Worst of Both Worlds

For most people with moderate to severe dry eye, aqueous tear-deficient dry eye and evaporative dry eye can actually coexist. When one of these types develops, no matter which affects the eyes first, the counterbalancing mechanism begins to work overtime to try to counteract the effects of the initial problem and stabilize the moisture content of your eyes. This compensatory reaction soon exhausts itself, which results in the second type of dry eye. The fact is that anyone who has moderate to severe dry eye is likely suffering from both aqueous tear-deficient dry eye and evaporative dry eye.

DEVELOPMENT OF DRY EYE

Because dry eye disease has a number of possible causes, the condition can develop in a number of possible ways. In its most common form, the front layer of the tear film, or the lipid layer, somehow breaks down. When this happens, some patients will complain that their vision fluctuates throughout the day and they need to continually blink to clear it. Other patients may complain that it becomes harder for them to read as the day goes on. Others may notice that their computer viewing becomes more difficult and that they need to take more breaks. In addition, in rare cases, some people may even experience dry eye during the middle of the night. (Yes, it is rare, but it happens.)

In some instances, patients don't even realize they have dry eye. The reason that there might be a discrepancy between having dry eye and the appearance of dry eye symptoms comes down to the nerves at the front of the eye. When they are not functioning properly, these nerves may not send the correct signals in connection with low levels of tears.

The number one demographic for dry eyes is women over forty years of age. Researchers have tried to explain why this group might be more susceptible to this disease, and the most likely culprit is hormones. It seems that there are hormone receptors on the tear glands, and as hormone levels change around the time of menopause, the production of tears may be altered as well.

Table 2.1. Dry Eye Symptoms

Condition	Symptoms	Complications
Mild	Scratchiness, burning, stinging, mild blurring of vision.	Reduction in contact lens tolerance, irritation-induced reflex tearing.
Moderate	Marked ocular discomfort, reduction in vision.	Reduction in antibacterial function of tear film, superficial punctate keratitis (a condition marked by painful, watery eyes that are sensitive to light. Blurring of vision, burning sensation, and the feeling of a foreign object being lodged in the eye may also occur).
Severe	Severe irritation, burning, blurring of vision.	Superficial punctate keratitis, filamentary keratitis (same symptoms as superficial punctate keratitis), secondary lid infections.

EFFECTS ON VISION

As outlined in Chapter 1, the cornea is the most forward part of the eye. While it is the first anatomical structure that light hits as it enter the eye, technically light must pass through the tear film, which coats the front of the cornea, on its way to the cornea.

As with all optical surfaces, uniformity is critical in maintaining a clear image to focus onto a focal point (in this case, the retina). While the cornea is a stable structure and can maintain its smooth optical surface, the tear film is a fluid and varies with each blink. Stability of the tear film presents a never-ending challenge for the visual system, but it is necessary for clear vision. Variations in the tear film, which include excessive tearing, dry spots, corneal irritation, etc., can lead to an unstable tear film, which can lead to visual distortions.

EFFECTS ON EYE HEALTH

The tear film fulfills several functions for the eye. As the cornea does not contain any blood vessels through which to receive nutrients, two of the most important functions of the tear film are to nourish the cornea and protect it from invading pathogens. The tear film supplies oxygen to the eye to maintain corneal cell health, proteins to support tear structure, enzymes to protect it against harmful molecules, and various antioxidants to prevent free radicals from damaging the ocular surface. More specifically, the tear film supplies helpful substances such as ascorbic acid, lactoferrin, amino acids, electrolytes, and immunoglobulins. Ascorbic acid, also known as vitamin C, is an important antioxidant. Lactoferrin works to stop bacteria and viruses from forming on the tear film. *Amino acids* are the building blocks of proteins, which support the tear structure and can be indicators of some diseases. Electrolytes assist in fluid balance within the tear film. Immunoglobulins are proteins that are used by the immune system to neutralize pathogens. The tear glands secrete these fluids to create the tear film.

Due to constant light exposure, the eye surface is particularly endangered by oxygen free radicals, which are induced by photochemical reactions. Photochemical reactions happen when light energy affects a molecule to generate a reactive process. Enzymes in the tear film are also enlisted to fight off invading organisms, which can affect corneal health.

The aqueous layer of the tears contains a complex mixture of proteins, mucins, and electrolytes, which not only nourish but also protect the eye's surface. If your eyes begin to dry for any reason, harmful proteins known as *cytokines* can enter your tears, changing their consistency. This change reduces the wetness of your tears and increases their salt concentration, thus drying your eyes. Because the cornea depends on tears for both nourishment and protection, it then becomes susceptible to irritation, injury, and disease. Most likely, the conjunctiva will experience inflammation, making your eyes more susceptible to conditions like pink eye, allergies, corneal infections, eyelid infections, and more.

FROM DRY EYE TO PINK EYE

Pink eye, or *conjunctivitis,* refers to inflammation of the covering of the eye and the lining of the inside of the eyelids, otherwise known as the conjunctiva. It is one of the most common eye conditions and can be extremely contagious. Unfortunately, having dry eye can make you more susceptible to getting pink eye. The aqueous layer of the tear film contains cells that help fight off infection. If this watery layer is compromised, the conjunctiva and cornea are more vulnerable to bacterial and viral infections, which can lead to pink eye. Pink eye is defined by symptoms such as redness in one or both eyes, a feeling of a foreign substance being lodged in one or both eyes, itchiness in one or both eyes, and discharge in one or both eyes that can form a crust overnight. Restoration of the tear film to its full strength is required to prevent future infection.

There are several forms of conjunctivitis, one of which is known as *allergic conjunctivitis.* This form stems from a reaction of the body to an allergen (usually airborne). In fact, because dry eye disease and allergies share many similar symptoms, dry eye disease and related conditions are often confused with allergies.

ALLERGIES OR DRY EYE?

While experts should be able to differentiate between allergy symptoms and symptoms of dry eye, it is understandable that the average person would be uncertain as to whether she was being tormented by dry eye disease or by hay fever. There are many similarities between the signs of allergies and the signs of dry eye, but a detailed list of each condition's main symptoms should help you figure out whether it is dry eye or allergies about which you should be complaining.

Some of the signs of an allergy are itchiness, swelling, puffiness, constant tearing, crusting with mucus, nasal congestion, sneezing, and itchy throat. Signs of dry eye include dryness in the eye, grittiness in the eye, sporadic tearing, lid crusting, ocular fatigue, and blepharitis (eyelid inflammation).

Spring and fall are often the most difficult times for allergy sufferers, although some may suffer year-round. Contact lenses may increase the intensity and duration of the allergic response, as allergens can become trapped under a lens or stick to its surface. If you have allergies, there may be times during the year when you are so uncomfortable that you cannot wear your contacts.

Now that you know the similarities and differences between allergy symptoms and symptoms of dry eye, you may find that you exhibit signs of both conditions. Your doctor should be able to look closely at your eyes and analyze the evidence to make a definitive diagnosis. Of course, if it is early spring and you find yourself sneezing and rubbing your eyes, there is good reason to suspect allergies as the cause of your eye troubles, and a good chance your doctor will confirm your suspicions.

CONCLUSION

It should now be apparent that dry eye disease is not as simple as it sounds. Not all dry eye patients respond with a complete reduction of symptoms after just one treatment. Dry eye is multifactorial, so not every case of dry eye is exactly the same, either in presentation or in response to treatment. Without understanding the true cause of the disease and the interaction of its confounding factors, a doctor will not be able to treat all dry eye patients effectively. The following chapter explores the factors that cause dry eye disease so that you, too, can have a voice in your treatment and play an informed role in the alleviation of your dry eye condition.

3

The Many Causes of Dry Eye

While the definition of dry eye disease is an evolving one, millions of people are suffering from this condition right now. In order to address a case of dry eye properly, a doctor must determine its cause. Of course, age is always a factor, as the eyes produce about 40 percent less moisture with advancing age. Nevertheless, many other conditions can contribute to dry eye, some more serious than others. Ultimately, as a dry eye patient, you simply want to be comfortable and see clearly again, and finding out what's behind your particular case of dry eye is the best way to resolve it with the right treatment.

AUTOIMMUNE DISEASE

Your immune system, which comprises infection-fighting components known as *white blood cells*, or *leukocytes*, protects your body from many different harmful substances. Under normal conditions, your immune system fights off only unwanted invaders, such as viruses and bacteria. If your immune system malfunctions, however, it can also attack normal cells in your body, making you sick. *Autoimmune disease* refers to a condition in which this abnormal immune reaction occurs in response to a normal part of the body. There are at least eighty types of autoimmune disease, and nearly any body part can be involved. Typical symptoms include low-grade fever and fatigue, although different forms of autoimmune disease can have much worse symptoms. Some common illnesses that are considered autoimmune diseases include celiac disease, diabetes, Graves' disease, Hashimoto's disease, inflammatory bowel disease, multiple sclerosis, psoriasis, rheumatoid arthritis, and lupus. Many autoimmune diseases have an effect on the eyes and can lead to dry eye.

Diabetes

Type 1 diabetes is an autoimmune disease that occurs when the body mistakenly sees its own insulin-producing cells, or *pancreatic beta cells*, as foreign invaders and destroys them. *Insulin* is a hormone that allows glucose, or sugar, to enter your cells and be used as an energy source. When you eat carbohydrates, your body breaks them down into *blood glucose,* or *blood sugar,* and without insulin, your blood sugar levels would be consistently elevated, which can damage blood vessels and organs over time.

Studies have shown a correlation between diabetes and dry eye. In fact, they suggest that the higher the HbA1c value, which refers to a long-term blood sugar reading, the greater the chance of dry eye. An HbA1c level below 5.7 percent is considered normal. An HbA1c between 5.7 and 6.4 percent signals prediabetes, and a reading of 6.5 and over is considered full-blown diabetes. Approximately half the diabetic population is afflicted with dry eye. Diabetes, however, can also lead to a loss of corneal sensation, so many diabetics do not know they have dry eye. The likelihood of a diabetic patient acquiring dry eye increases with age, and diabetes-associated dry eye is 50 percent more common in female patients than in male patients. Unfortunately, the exact mechanism that causes dry eye in diabetics is not fully understood.

Dysfunction in the autonomic nervous system seems to contribute to the problem. The autonomic nervous system acts largely unconsciously and regulates bodily functions such as heart rate, digestion, respiratory rate, pupillary response, urination, sexual arousal, and tear production. Diabetes-related nerve damage can hinder proper communication between the brain and other organs and the autonomic nervous system, resulting in poor tear function, among other problems.

The surface of the eye is one of the most sensitive tissues in the body and can be easily damaged by the physiological changes caused by diabetes, leading to a loss of sensation in the cornea, as previously mentioned. This loss of corneal sensation not only makes dry eye harder for diabetics to recognize but also breaks the feedback mechanism that monitors tear levels. As a result, production of tears drops significantly and the eyes dry out. Unfortunately, this outcome makes diabetics prone to conjunctivitis and inflammation of the eyelid margin, which also lead to dry eye.

In addition, as diabetes progresses, it can damage the small blood vessels that feed oxygen to the front of the eye. When these vessels become fragile, they also become less able to deliver an adequate supply of oxygen to the eye, without which it cannot function normally. Finally, dysfunction of the meibomian glands within the eyelids has been associated with diabetes and can lead to a loss of tears. This type of dysfunction has also been found in connection with lupus, another autoimmune disease that can cause dry eye.

In type 2 diabetes, your body is unable to use insulin properly and thus cannot absorb glucose from your bloodstream. Linked to excess weight and inactivity, this form of diabetes is not considered an autoimmune disease, although recent studies suggest it may have an autoimmune component. Whether or not it is ever categorized as a true autoimmune disease, type 2 diabetes, like type 1 diabetes, can lead to dry eye. This information is worth noting, as approximately 95 percent of diabetics suffer from type 2.

Lupus

Systemic lupus erythematosus (SLE), more commonly known as lupus, is a chronic autoimmune disease that exhibits a wide range of symptoms due to its impact on virtually every organ. While the most common symptoms of lupus include fever, joint pain, and rash, dry eye disease is the most likely symptom in the eye. Antibodies produced in the bloodstream of lupus patients can affect the skin, heart, lungs, kidneys, joints, nervous system, and eyes, where they can be deposited in many eye tissues. Deposited antibodies in the conjunctiva, cornea, or lacrimal glands can reduce tear production and deplete the mucin layer of the tear film. In addition, lupus can cause changes in blood vessels in the eye and inflammation of the inner and outer layers of the eye, which can affect the lacrimal glands in the conjunctiva, reducing tear production.

Approximately 20 percent of lupus patients also develop secondary Sjögren's syndrome (see page 27). This condition is characterized by arthritis, dry mouth, tingling sensation , and dry eye syndrome due to the lacrimal glands' inability to produce enough tears to lubricate the eyes properly, which results in a feeling of itchiness, grittiness, or burning in the eyes.

Lupus has also been linked to meibomian gland dysfunction, which can lead to a weak lipid layer of the tear film. When this layer has been depleted of oil, tears evaporate too quickly. Finally, even if lupus is being managed adequately with medications, some of the medications used in the treatment of this autoimmune disease can have negative effects on your eye health.

Ocular Rosacea

Rosacea is a chronic skin condition of the facial area. It is characterized by symptoms such as facial flushing, skin redness, spider veins, skin coarseness, and inflammatory eruption of the skin similar to acne. Although rosacea is not an autoimmune disease, increasing evidence suggests a link between this condition and autoimmune disease.

Rosacea affects approximately 14 million Americans, and of those affected, about 60 percent experience associated eye complications, known as *ocular rosacea.*

Symptoms of ocular rosacea include redness, burning, stinging, and irritation of the eye, as well as the feeling of a foreign substance in the eye. Ocular rosacea can also lead to swollen eyelids due to inflammation of the meibomian glands, also known as *blepharitis.* This meibomian gland dysfunction results in an increase in the rate of evaporation of tears, which causes dry eye.

Rheumatoid Arthritis

Rheumatoid arthritis (RA) is an autoimmune disease that causes pain, stiffness, swelling, and loss of function in the joints. Although it is the most common type of autoimmune arthritis, its development is still not completely understood. Rheumatoid arthritis can also damage your skin, eyes, lungs, heart, kidneys, salivary glands, nerve tissue, bone marrow, and blood vessels. In fact, almost half of all rheumatoid arthritis sufferers experience symptoms in these bodily structures.

Rheumatoid arthritis, like lupus, can eventually lead to secondary Sjögren's syndrome, which, as explained in the next section, is associated with a deficiency in tear production. If you have RA, you have a 25 percent chance of experiencing dry eye.

Sjögren's Syndrome

Although *Sjögren's syndrome* (pronounced "SHOW-grins" syndrome) impacts the entire body, the moisture-producing glands in the eyes and mouth are typically affected first, as small white blood cells called *lymphocytes* attack the lacrimal (eye) and salivary (mouth) glands. Once damaged, these glands can no longer produce tears or saliva, and eye and mouth dryness result. When the sinuses, skin, and vaginal tissues are affected, dryness occurs in these places as well.

Although Sjögren's patients predominantly experience its major symptoms, which include dry eye, dry mouth, fatigue, and joint pain, this autoimmune disease can also cause dysfunction of the kidneys, gastrointestinal system, blood vessels, lungs, liver, pancreas, or central nervous system, and lymph node tumors. As many as four million Americans are living with this disease, with nine out of ten patients being women.

Thyroid Disease

The thyroid gland makes and stores hormones that affect every cell in the body. These hormones help regulate important biological functions, including heart rate, blood pressure, body temperature, and metabolism (the rate at which food is converted into energy). Thyroid hormones also help regulate brain development, growth, muscle control, digestive function, and even mood.

Dysfunction of the thyroid gland typically presents as an overactive thyroid, known as *hyperthyroidism,* or and underactive thyroid, known as *hypothyroidism.* In hyperthyroidism, the thyroid releases too much hormone, which leads to symptoms of fatigue, weakness, tremor, weight loss, heat intolerance, and enlargement of the thyroid. The autoimmune disease known as Graves' disease is the most common form of hyperthyroidism, and the type of thyroid disease that affects the eyes most. The course of hyperthyroidism leads to a condition in which the eyes bulge forward. This bulging, typically caused by a thickening of eye muscles behind the eyes, prevents the eyelids from closing properly, and therefore creates a dry eye condition.

The autoimmune disease known as Hashimoto's disease is the most common form of hypothyroidism, in which the thyroid produces less than a sufficient amount of hormones. Symptoms of this disease include constipation, pale, dry skin, weight gain, and muscle or joint stiffness and pain. Enlargement of the thyroid, called *goiter,* is also often seen. Hashimoto's disease is about eight times more common in women, and eye signs include a decrease in tear production and an increase in tear evaporation.

COMPUTER USE

While it has lead to many positive developments, the information age has also created a challenge to the surface of the eye. From desktop computers, which changed the way we view documents, to laptops, cell phones, and tablets, which allow us to view anything we need (or want) to view at practically anytime, our eyes are not adapting well to this new screen-based technology.

Originally, computer monitors were set on workplace desks in a fixed position. Workers had to adjust their body postures to this new position in order to view their documents, which were now being displayed in a vertical position (screen) rather than a horizontal one (desk). Viewing a document on a traditionally placed computer monitor requires the eyelids to be more open than they would be if the viewer were looking down at a desk to view a document. Due to this larger eyelid opening, normal blinking becomes more difficult, which leads to eye dryness, of course.

Studies have also shed light on other technology-related issues that can lead to dry eye. They have shown that computer users do not blink as often as non-users, and that their blinking is not as complete as it should be. Both situations can lead to excessive evaporation of tears.

Kids and Dry Eye

It is likely that most people who pick up this book will be over forty years old, for the simple reason that most people who experience dry eye are over forty. In recent years, however, doctors have been seeing younger and younger patients with this condition. Given the amount of time kids spend looking at cell phones and tablets, it should not be surprising that their eyes become stressed in many ways.

A study performed at the Pacific University College of Optometry showed that, given two different viewing conditions (paper-based vs. screen-based), students held the screen closer than the paper for the same size font. It was not determined why this occurred, but it is almost universally acknowledged that kids stare at near-viewing tasks more closely, more intensely, and for longer periods than do adults.

Then there are video games. If you have children under the age of thirty, you have likely witnessed how addictive these games can be. Studies on video game users show they hardly ever blink! It seems that blinking would cause a loss of concentration (however briefly), so gamers stare incessantly at the screen, trying to maintain their concentration. It is not surprising that dry eye would be a consequence of this behavior.

And we should not forget the sociological and environmental aspects of how we use our eyes on a daily basis. Whereas early man (cavemen) likely only used their daytime vision for survival (making weapons, hunting, fishing, etc.) and slept as the sun went down, we now can be productive in our society for almost twenty-four hours a day. The dawn of the electronic age has ushered in an unprecedented use of our eyes for near-point activities, which dominates our viewing time. Over-focusing at near-viewing targets (reading text, video screens) and the desire to take in more information lead to a "wide-open" viewing posture for our eyes, therefore demanding a stronger tear film that can maintain its integrity for longer periods. The tear film has not adjusted to the increased demand, thus will weaken and break down sooner, creating a dry eye condition.

CONTACT LENSES

Millions of people successfully wear contact lenses, with over 80 percent of them wearing some form of soft lens. Whenever a lens is placed directly on the eye (the cornea, specifically) the tear layer becomes split between the front and back surface of the lens. Because of this division, each of these tear layers is thinner than the original tear film. These thinner tear layers can break down, leading to dry spots over the soft contact lens material.

As wearing time increases, proteins and other elements in the tear film can deposit themselves onto these dry spots. This creates an expanding area of dryness on the lens, which explains the increasing dryness contact lens wearers feel as the day progresses. If lenses are not cleaned properly, these deposits can become embedded in them, continuing to contribute to the dry lens experience of the wearer day after day.

When discussing contact lenses with patients, eye doctors often ask about "end of day" comfort, the level of which can indicate a potential dry eye condition. Adding lubrication drops to contact lenses may help prevent dryness to some degree, but these drops are often needed several times a day, which can interfere with a person's lifestyle and comfort.

What most patients do not realize is that there are dozens of different types of soft contact lenses made of various materials. When it comes to dry eye, focus should be placed on a material's moisture content. The original soft lenses (circa 1970) were made of a material called HEMA. At the time, this material was revolutionary for its hydrophilic, or "water-loving," quality, which made contact lenses quite compatible with the surface of the eye. The lenses, however, were meant to last an entire year, so cleaning and disinfecting them was a major concern. Even with this helpful new material, it was challenging to maintain comfort and eye health as a wearer of contact lenses.

Updated lens materials (notably silicone hydrogel), design, and maintenance methods have led to lenses that are better for long-term wear and more economical to manufacture. It has also led to the "daily disposable" lens category as the ultimate in comfort and convenience. No matter the lenses, however, they still split your tear film into two layers and can cause discomfort if your tear film is not fully formed and stable. At the end of the day, the more compatible a type of contact lens is with your tear film, the less chance it has of causing dry eye.

CORNEAL DISEASE

Given that the back layer of the tear film adheres to the corneal surface, any disease or disorder of the cornea can lead to dry eye. When it comes to determining the cause of your dry eye, the following corneal conditions should be considered as possible candidates.

Foreign Body/Scratched Cornea

This is the most common malady of the cornea. The corneal surface is naturally soft and moist. Its cells allow it to be transparent, providing clear vision. Any foreign body that can scrape the corneal surface or lodge under the eyelid can lead to a corneal abrasion, or scratched cornea. Fortunately, the cornea is a fast-healing structure, so it typically replaces its damaged cells with new ones within twenty-four hours. Temporary dryness, however, is certainly a common effect of this issue.

Keratitis

The root word "kerato" refers to the cornea and any "itis" describes an inflammation. Yet inflammation of the cornea, or *keratitis,* is different than inflammation anywhere else in the body due to the lack of blood vessels in this structure. An inflammation of the cornea will not allow the tear film to anchor itself properly to the front surface cells, resulting in pain, irritation, and dryness.

Recurrent Corneal Erosion

As its name indicates, *recurrent corneal erosion* refers to a wearing away of corneal cells, typically caused by a trauma or genetic defect. The symptom of pain in the morning is the most common, due to cells rubbing away from the cornea upon awakening. Because the front surface of the cornea is irregular in this condition, drying of the surface is also a common symptom.

DEMODEX

As previously explained, many cases of dry eye emanate from a disruption of the integrity of the tear film due to an inflammation or infection of the eyelids. A significant—but rarely considered—condition of the eyelids is an infestation of a microscopic mite called *Demodex*. *Demodex* is a genus of tiny mites that live in or near hair follicles of mammals.

Two species live on humans: *Demodex folliculorum* and *Demodex brevis*, both frequently referred to as eyelash mites. Detection of these mites requires careful examination under high magnification. Difficult to treat, these mites can cause an eyelid reaction that affects the secretions of the meibomian glands and therefore leads to symptoms of dry eye.

ENVIRONMENT

Yet another factor that can have a significant effect on your level of tears is your environment. As your eyes are in direct contact with your external environment every day of your life, air quality matters. High elevations (e.g., Denver) or desert environments (e.g., Phoenix) have air humidity that is drier and can cause even "normal" eyes to feel dry. This goes for indoor environments as well. When using air-conditioning during the summer or heat during the winter, forced air circulation can exacerbate a marginal dry eye condition and turn it into a severe case. Air movement around your eyes (fans, open windows, etc.) can also lead to a drying of the eye surface, so check around your internal environment to see if you can control any drafts.

EYE SURGERY

Any time there is a "break" in the front part of the eye, which typically occurs in eye surgery, there is a disruption of the tear film. How well the tear film recovers and how long that recovery takes is dependent on how severe or intense the disruption of the tear film was and on the quality of the tear film prior to the procedure. This is true for just about every type of eye surgery.

In cataract surgery, the cornea is opened by an incision that can be anywhere from 3 to 15 millimeters long. Once the lens inside the eye has been removed (and replaced with an artificial lens), the cornea is sutured back together. Sometimes the surgeon will use self-dissolving sutures, or, if the incision is small enough, there may be no need for sutures. In either case, the nerves of the cornea are severed and it will take some time for them to grow back. These nerves supply feedback to the brain, which must readjust the tearing level.

Oxidative Stress

In addition, research has also shown that oxidative stress can have a profound effect on the ocular surface. Oxidative stress is caused by an imbalance between the production of reactive oxygen and a biological system's ability to detoxify the reactive molecules readily or repair the resulting damage easily. Oxidative stress has been shown to be involved in the development of dry eye disease. Increases in oxidative stress markers, changes in antioxidant-related gene expression, and decreased capacity of corneal epithelial cells in dry eye conditions suggest a relationship between the accumulation of oxidative stress and the development of corneal epithelial alterations.

A similar situation happens during LASIK surgery, which refers to laser vision correction, except that the cornea is not penetrated fully. Instead, a flap is created in the front layers of the cornea in order to allow the laser to remove some of the middle layers of the cornea, resulting in a flattening of the curvature of the cornea. Sutures are not used, allowing the flap to grow back and connect with the uncut cornea over time. While there are no sutures used in LASIK surgery, nerves are still severed, and a typical post-LASIK symptom is eye dryness. Most studies show that LASIK-related dry eye symptoms last approximately one year after the procedure.

Surgeons should test for dry eye disease before any surgical procedure. A preoperative dry eye condition can lead to an extended healing time, as many of the eye's healing factors are in the tear film. Be sure to ask your surgeon about this issue if you are thinking about eye surgery.

EYELID ISSUES

The eyelid is responsible for many important functions around the eye. Its main function is to protect the eye from environmentally related injury. This may be why the blink reflex is the fastest reflex in the body. Yet another important function of the eyelid is to clean the eye surface while the tear film spreads a new layer of tears onto the front of the eye and supplies nutrition to the cornea. If the edges of your eyelids are not even, uniform, and situated appropriately on the surface of your eye, your tears will not spread evenly. This can cause an irregularity in the thickness of your tear film, causing distortion of vision. Additionally, this inconsistency in your tear film can cause areas of thinning of the tear layer, leading to dry spots.

Eyelids are also susceptible to conditions such as blepharitis, which, as previously explained, is an inflammation of the eyelids that is associated with swelling, soreness, and a host of other symptoms, including those of dry eye. Many times, blepharitis is treated in the same manner as simple dry eye. When dry eye is caused by blepharitis, however, it can lead to excessive tearing, as tear glands attempt to compensate for the dryness by flushing the eye with tears. This is not always the case with dry eye, so blepharitis must be treated in a particular way, which is to address eyelid inflammation specifically.

Going along with the disease aspect of eyelids is the fact that women use cosmetics, which might play a role in dry eye disease. There may be toxins in many cosmetics, but the location in which these cosmetics are applied can also make a difference. A common location to apply eyeliner is the waterline of the eyelid, just inside the lower eyelashes. Unfortunately, this is where the pores of the meibomian glands are located, and applying a thick layer of eyeliner over these pores will not allow the meibomian oils to reach the tear film. Women should be conscious of this and apply eyeliner only on the "skin side" of the lower (and upper) eyelashes.

HORMONES

The demographic most affected by dry eye is women over forty years of age. When we think of the changes that occur with aging, alteration of hormone levels is one of the most significant, and especially for women. Lacrimal glands have hormone receptors located on their cells, so changes in hormone levels (as occurs in menopause) can alter the production of tears, but knowledge of the role of hormones in dry eye is still evolving.

The closest layer of the tear film to the cornea, the mucin layer contains mucin proteins, which are responsible for the slimy texture of mucus and give this layer its name. The cells that secrete these proteins are located in the cornea and conjunctiva and respond to hormonal stimulation. Therefore, anything that can affect hormone production may also affect the mucin layer of the tear film.

Estrogen has been shown to decrease lipid production, which may be the link between dry eye and hormone replacement therapy (HRT). This relationship, however, does not provide a good explanation for why postmenopausal women have a higher prevalence of dry eye. The association is not clearly understood, but it may be due to a decrease in testosterone activity on the meibomian glands. Testosterone is an androgen hormone, and androgen hormones are known to increase lipid production in sebaceous glands. In light of this information, it would be reasonable to expect meibomian glands to be more active in the presence of higher levels of testosterone as well. Currently, testosterone is thought to be protective against dry eye through its effects on both meibomian and lacrimal glands.

Often physicians will prescribe hormone replacement therapy to ease symptoms associated with the transition to menopause. HRT is somewhat controversial, though, and may be linked to elevated risks of endometrial cancer, heart attack, and stroke, despite being protective against the effects of osteoporosis.

Most research regarding HRT and the eye has been directed towards dry eye disease. Early studies concluded that women using HRT actually had a decrease in eye symptoms but later studies suggested that women using HRT experienced a 30 to 70 percent increase in the development of dry eye. In general, HRT is not detrimental to eye health but those who are on this therapy and experience dry eye should share this information with their eyecare practitioners.

INFLAMMATION

While we know inflammation is one of the mechanisms that cause damage to the ocular surface in dry eye disease, the role of inflammation in dry eye is not completely understood. The entire inflammatory process is a complicated one throughout the body. From a treatment point of view, however, the inflammatory process has a lot of entry points that can be attacked. In other words, there are many different points along the process that are vulnerable to different kinds of therapeutic agents such as drugs that interfere with the process of inflammation. Therefore, inflammation is a very attractive target for investigators and companies developing new drugs.

In the evaporative form of dry eye, the surface of the eye becomes exposed to a concentrated high-salt solution. This can destroy the cells on the cornea's surface, which then elicits an inflammatory response. Inflammation can lead to dysfunction of tear secretion, which then increases the salt concentration even more. In addition, as previously mentioned, some dry eye sufferers also have autoimmune diseases, in which inflammation plays a primary role in disrupting the function of lacrimal glands.

MEDICATIONS

Pharmaceuticals are used to treat medical conditions, but they often come with side effects, which can affect different parts of the body, including the tear film. Medications that can cause dry eye include diuretics (commonly used to treat high blood pressure), antihistamines and decongestants (allergy and sinus treatments), sleeping pills, birth control pills, antidepressants, drugs for acne treatment, gastric medications (such as those for irritable bowel syndrome) and opiate-based pain relievers, such as morphine. Since allergies are among the most common health conditions, antihistamines are the leading contributor to dry eye in terms of medications.

The average American adult over the age of fifty takes about seven medications to address various health issues. No medication is without side effects, and many medications, in fact, are dispensed to treat side effects of other medications. Thus, it is not at all surprising that the production and stability of the tear film could be affected by some of these medications.

NUTRITIONAL DEFICIENCY

The tissues in the front of the eye are very susceptible to nutritional deficiencies. The cell type that makes up the front surface of the cornea and conjunctiva is the epithelial cell. Vitamin A is critical in maintaining the moisture of this cell, thus a vitamin A deficiency will negatively affect the cornea and conjunctiva, creating a dry eye environment. Fortunately, vitamin A deficiency is rare in the United States.

Tear film integrity is very much dependent on the lipid layer, and the consistency of the lipid layer is dependent on the body's ability to process fatty acids, such as omega-3 and omega-6 fatty acids. When this process is disrupted in any way, dry eye can result. The role of fatty acids in maintaining the integrity of the tear film is discussed in greater detail in Chapter 6 along with other nutritional approaches to the treatment of dry eye. (See page 65.)

SLEEP DISORDERS

It should come as no surprise that your body requires a sufficient amount of restful sleep in order to function properly. Insufficient sleep has been linked to many chronic health problems, including depression, obesity, type 2 diabetes, cardiovascular disease, and even dry eye disease. Research has shown that quality of sleep can play a role in the development of dry eye disease. A number of studies have drawn a connection between sleep disorders such as sleep apnea and dry eye disease.

Of course, after a long day of using your eyes, they are naturally dried out. It makes sense that a sleep disorder such as insomnia would lead to dry eye, as it causes your eyes to remain in use for an even longer time because you are awake for much of the night as well. Moreover, there may be other connections between nighttime and dry eye. For example, metabolism slows during sleep. As body functions slow, so does blood circulation, which causes fewer nutrients to reach the eye and fewer tears to be produced.

CONCLUSION

There are so many possible causes of dry eye that it may seem as though almost anything could lead to this condition. Dry eye can be a result of health problems, lifestyle, dietary choices, environmental conditions, or some combination of these factors. If you are experiencing dryness around your eyes or they tend to tear often, then you likely have dry eye and need some assistance, whatever the cause of it may be.

There are a handful of tests available to help your eye doctor diagnose dry eye, which the following chapter describes in detail.

4

$\mathscr{T}$esting for Dry Eye

lthough it might seem otherwise, identifying dry eye is not always an easy task. Sometimes doctors see patients who complain of eye dryness and exhibit the typical symptoms of dry eye disease. Other times, patients will have dry eye but not even know it, which presents a challenge to their doctors. This chapter looks at the different tests doctors perform in order to diagnose dry eye disease in a patient. These examinations include patient questionnaires and medical procedures, both of which are meant to provide a doctor with the information required to make a determination. Knowing a little bit about the tests you are asked to undergo will give you a better sense of what your doctor is looking for and why.

PATIENT QUESTIONNAIRES

While doctors can perform all sorts of medical tests to diagnose a condition such as dry eye, they often start by taking a statement from the patient in the form of a questionnaire. Fortunately, when it comes to dry eye, there are several questionnaires available that can give your doctor a good sense of the dry eye symptoms you are experiencing. The three most popular are the Ocular Surface Disease Index (OSDI), the Dry Eye Questionnaire 5 (DEQ-5), and the Standardized Patient Evaluation of Eye Dryness (SPEED) survey.

Ocular Surface Disease Index (OSDI)

The Ocular Surface Disease Index (OSDI) is a questionnaire that provides an assessment of a patient's dry eye symptoms. (See Figure 4.1 on pages 41 and 42.) To develop this questionnaire, researchers distributed questions to over 400 patients with dry eye disease, who were asked to indicate whether they were experiencing any of the symptoms or problems on the list and, if so, how often. They narrowed down the list to twelve questions, which proved to be the most pertinent to an accurate assessment of dry eye. A score of 33 to 100 indicates dry eye disease, with higher scores corresponding to more severe cases.

Dry Eye Questionnaire 5 (DEQ-5)

The Dry Eye Questionnaire 5 (DEQ-5) was developed by Dr. Carolyn Begley et al. of Indiana University and designed to facilitate dry eye diagnosis and distinguish between different levels of severity of dry eye disease. (See Figure 4.2 on page 43.) The DEQ-5 questionnaire is short (it contains only five questions, as its name suggests), and compiles scores for frequency and late-day intensity of eye discomfort, frequency and late-day intensity of eye dryness, and frequency of watery eyes, totaling these scores at the end of the questionnaire. The DEQ-5 is very effective at discriminating between normal subjects and subjects with dry eye. A score of 6 or greater indicates dry eye and a score over 12 suggests a possible diagnosis of Sjögren's syndrome.

Standardized Patient Evaluation of Eye Dryness (SPEED)

The Standardized Patient Evaluation of Eye Dryness (SPEED) questionnaire was developed by TearScience, Inc. (See Figure 4.3 on page 44.) It evaluates both the frequency and severity of dry eye symptoms. It relies on a scale of 0 to 3 for patients to rate the frequency of their symptoms, with 0 being "never" and 3 being "constant." It relies on a scale of 0 to 4 for patients to rate the severity of their symptoms, with 0 being "no problems" and 4 being "intolerable" symptoms. The total score, which can range from 0 to 28, is a sum of the scores for each answer. The questions are designed to elicit responses regarding the patient's symptoms currently and over the previous three months.

Ocular Surface Disease Index© (OSDI©)[2]

Ask your patients the following 12 questions, and circle the number in the box that best represents each answer. Then, fill in boxes A, B, C, D, and E according to the instructions beside each.

Have you experienced any of the following *during the last week*?	All of the time	Most of the time	Half of the time	Some of the time	None of the time
1. Eyes that are sensitive to light? . .	4	3	2	1	0
2. Eyes that feel gritty?	4	3	2	1	0
3. Painful or sore eyes?	4	3	2	1	0
4. Blurred vision?	4	3	2	1	0
5. Poor vision?	4	3	2	1	0

Subtotal score for answers 1 to 5   (A)

Have problems with your eyes limited you in performing any of the following *during the last week*?	All of the time	Most of the time	Half of the time	Some of the time	None of the time	N/A
6. Reading?	4	3	2	1	0	N/A
7. Driving at night?	4	3	2	1	0	N/A
8. Working with a computer or bank machine (ATM)?	4	3	2	1	0	N/A
9. Watching TV?	4	3	2	1	0	N/A

Subtotal score for answers 6 to 9   (B)

Have your eyes felt uncomfortable in any of the following situations *during the last week*?	All of the time	Most of the time	Half of the time	Some of the time	None of the time	N/A
10. Windy conditions?	4	3	2	1	0	N/A
11. Places or areas with low humidity (very dry)?	4	3	2	1	0	N/A
12. Areas that are air conditioned? . . .	4	3	2	1	0	N/A

Subtotal score for answers 10 to 12   (C)

Add subtotals A, B, and C to obtain D
(D = sum of scores for all questions answered)   (D)

Total number of questions answered
(do not include questions answered N/A)   (E)

Please turn over the questionnaire to calculate the patient's final OSDI° score.

Figure 4.1. Ocular Surface Disease Index.

Evaluating the OSDI© Score[1]

The OSDI© is assessed on a scale of 0 to 100, with higher scores representing greater disability. The index demonstrates sensitivity and specificity in distinguishing between normal subjects and patients with dry eye disease. The OSDI© is a valid and reliable instrument for measuring dry eye disease (normal, mild to moderate, and severe) and effect on vision-related function.

Assessing Your Patient's Dry Eye Disease[1, 2]

Use your answers D and E from side 1 to compare the sum of scores for all questions answered (D) and the number of questions answered (E) with the chart below.* Find where your patient's score would fall. Match the corresponding shade of red to the key below to determine whether your patient's score indicates normal, mild, moderate, or severe dry eye disease.

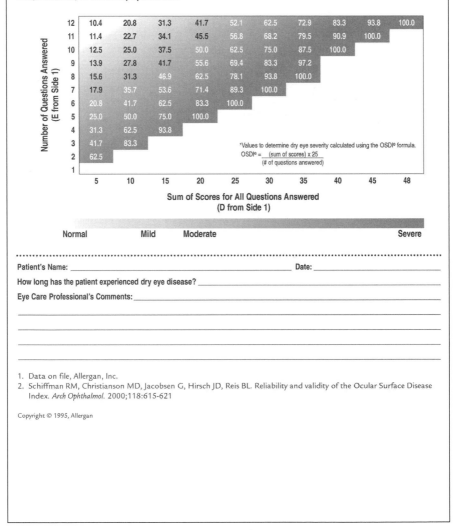

1. Data on file, Allergan, Inc.
2. Schiffman RM, Christianson MD, Jacobsen G, Hirsch JD, Reis BL. Reliability and validity of the Ocular Surface Disease Index. *Arch Ophthalmol.* 2000;118:615-621

Figure 4.1 cont'd. Ocular Surface Disease Index.

DEQ 5

1. Questions about **EYE DISCOMFORT**:
   a. During a typical day in the past month, **how often** did your eyes feel discomfort?

   0 Never
   1 Rarely
   2 Sometimes
   3 Frequently
   4 Constantly

   b. When your eyes felt discomfort, **how intense was this feeling of discomfort** at the end of the day, within two hours of going to bed?

Never have it	Not at All Intense				Very Intense
0	**1**	**2**	**3**	**4**	**5**

2. Questions about **EYE DRYNESS**:
   a. During a typical day in the past month, **how often** did your eyes feel dry?

   0 Never
   1 Rarely
   2 Sometimes
   3 Frequently
   4 Constantly

   b. When your eyes felt dry, **how intense was this feeling of dryness** at the end of the day, within two hours of going to bed?

Never have it	Not at All Intense				Very Intense
0	**1**	**2**	**3**	**4**	**5**

3. Question about **WATERY EYES**:
   During a typical day in the past month, **how often** did your eyes look or feel excessively watery?

   0 Never
   1 Rarely
   2 Sometimes
   3 Frequently
   4 Constantly

   Score: 1a + 1b + 2a + 2b + 3 = Total
   ___ + ___ + ___ + ___ + ___ = _____

Figure 4.2. Dry Eye Questionnaire 5.

SPEED™ QUESTIONNAIRE

Name: _____ Date: ___/___/___ Sex: M F (Circle) DOB: ___/___/___

For the Standardized Patient Evaluation of Eye Dryness (SPEED) Questionnaire, please answer the following questions by checking the box that best represents your answer. Select only one answer per question.

1. Report the type of SYMPTOMS you experience and when they occur:

Symptoms	At this visit		Within past 72 hours		Within past 3 months	
	Yes	No	Yes	No	Yes	No
Dryness, Grittiness or Scratchiness						
Soreness or Irritation						
Burning or Watering						
Eye Fatigue						

2. Report the FREQUENCY of your symptoms using the rating list below:

Symptoms	0	1	2	3
Dryness, Grittiness or Scratchiness				
Soreness or Irritation				
Burning or Watering				
Eye Fatigue				

0 = Never **1** = Sometimes **2** = Often **3** = Constant

3. Report the SEVERITY of your symptoms using the rating list below:

Symptoms	0	1	2	3	4
Dryness, Grittiness or Scratchiness					
Soreness or Irritation					
Burning or Watering					
Eye Fatigue					

0 = No Problems
1 = Tolerable - not perfect, but not uncomfortable
2 = Uncomfortable - irritating, but does not interfere with my day
3 = Bothersome - irritating and interferes with my day
4 = Intolerable - unable to perform my daily tasks

4. Do you use eye drops for lubrication? ☐ YES ☐ NO If yes, how often? _____

Cornea. 2013 Sep;32(9):1204-10
13-ADV-123 A

For office use only
Total SPEED score (Frequency + Severity) = ___/28

Figure 4.3. Standardized Patient Evaluation of Eye Dryness.

Like the OSDI, the SPEED questionnaire is a useful tool in the diagnosis of dry eye, but its results should not be considered in lieu of findings from the OSDI. Research suggests that the SPEED questionnaire's values correlate best with the measurements of evaporative dry eye, while the OSDI's values correlate best with measurements of aqueous tear-deficient dry eye. Nevertheless, a diagnosis of evaporative or aqueous tear-deficient dry eye cannot be based solely on the results of these questionnaires.

MEDICAL TESTS

This book is not designed to teach you how to be an eye doctor, but it is meant to provide a basic understanding of some of the medical tests for dry eye a doctor might request. By comprehending the information attained from each test, you will be able to have more fruitful discussions with your doctor than you may have otherwise, which may raise your chance of successful treatment and recovery.

Tear Break-Up Time (TBUT)

As you are now well aware, the stability of the tear film is dependent on the integrity of its front layer, the lipid layer. Doctors test the stability of this layer adding a dye to the tear film and illuminating this dye with a blue light, making it glow bright green. As the patient blinks, the dye in the tear film spreads across the eye, creating an evenly distributed bright green-colored tear film. The eye must then remain open for an extended period of time, during which the doctor observes this green layer of tears until black areas appear in the green tear layer, which indicate that the tear film has begun to break down. The doctor records the number of seconds that elapse between the last blink and the appearance of the first dry spot. The result is known as the *tear break-up time* (TBUT). A TBUT under ten seconds is considered indicative of dry eye.

Noninvasive Keratograph Tear Break-Up Time (NIK-TBUT)

Some children may be reluctant to have a dye placed in their eyes. Unlike the use of dilating drops, the use of dye requires more cooperation from the patient. The *keratograph* is a device that uses infrared illumination to measure tear break-up time noninvasively, without the need to use any dye. Patients are simply required to keep still for fifteen to twenty seconds while looking into this diagnostic instrument.

Schirmer's Test

Named after German ophthalmologist Otto Schirmer, *Schirmer's test* has been used for over a century. In this simple examination, a paper strip is inserted into the space between the eyeball and the lower eyelid for several minutes to measure the production of tears. Both eyes are tested at the same time. The patient's eyes must remain closed for five minutes, which some may consider a drawback of the procedure. Schirmer's test measures total tear secretion (basal and reflex tears), although sometimes a topical anesthetic is placed on the eye to ensure only basal tear secretion is measured.

After the five-minute mark, the paper is removed from each eye and the amount of moisture present on each strip is measured. A reading of more than 10 mm of moisture on the paper strip after 5 minutes is indicative of normal tear production. (Both eyes normally release the same amount of tears.) A reading of less than 10 mm is indicative of a low level of tear production, while a measurement of less than 5 mm is suggestive of severe dry eye.

These days, the use of Schirmer's test is somewhat controversial, with some doctors finding the test too inconsistent with actual clinical determinations to act as a diagnostic aid. In other words, a patient with a low Schirmer's score may not display symptoms of dry eye at all, while a patient with a normal reading may show obvious signs of dry eye. Many doctors, however, still find it a useful tool when used in combination with other diagnostic tests, such as TBUT.

Meibomian Gland Evaluation

When attempting to diagnose dry eye, the evaluation of meibomian gland function can be a valuable tool. It can determine the presence and severity of *meibomian gland dysfunction* (MGD), which causes tears to evaporate too quickly, making it a leading cause of dry eye. To test meibomian gland function, doctors apply consistent pressure along the eyelid margin to see if glands are expressing oil properly. They may do so using something as simple as a cotton swab or a medical device such as a speculum with a curved blade, which is pressed on the inner eyelid.

The Future of Tear Testing

When you go for your annual check-up, your doctor takes fluid samples—most commonly blood and urine. These fluids contain certain proteins that can indicate the presence of various diseases. Scientists are starting to realize that another bodily fluid can offer additional information (in the form of proteins) about your overall health: your tears. Research has shown that there may be up to 2,000 different proteins in the tears, and scientists are working on a protocol for detecting them. Currently, TearScan (see page 49) can test for the presence of lactoferrin (which can determine dry eye) or IgE (which can detect an allergic reaction). The procedure requires a technician to take a small sample of tears and feed this sample into the TearScan machine, which produces results in just a few minutes.

In connection with this type of testing, the future may be even more exciting. Scientists are now looking for other diagnostic proteins in tears and developing a new series of tests to detect each of these unique substances. For example, right now, a blood sample is used to measure a protein known as a prostate specific antigen, or PSA, which is an indicator of prostate cancer at certain levels. As PSA is similar to a type of protein found in tears, in the coming years, doctors might be able to detect prostate cancer using a tear sample instead. If so, then other types of cancer might be able to be found by the same method. This means that you could one day go to your eye doctor for an eye exam and be screened for possible cancers at the same time.

Ocular Surface Interferometer

The ocular surface interferometer is a popular technology used to test for the underlying causes of dry eye. The ocular surface interferometer known as the LipiView II is a noninvasive device that takes an accurate digital picture of a patient's tear film, allowing a doctor to determine if lipid deficiency is responsible for a patient's dry eye condition. The patient is asked to look directly at a special light camera and blink normally while a computer-aided program takes the necessary measurements that will reveal the lipid content and quality of the patient's tear film. The doctor then analyzes the results and determines the best course of action in terms of dry eye treatment.

TearLab

When the right balance of water and salt in the tear film is disrupted, dry eye generally follows. This balance is known as *osmolarity* (the saltiness of tears) and can be tested using a device known as TearLab. As the osmolarity level of your tears increases, the corneal surface cells become damaged. For this test, your doctor will need an amount of tear fluid no larger than the period at the end of this sentence. The doctor or technician will take a tear sample from the corner of your eye (this is painless). The sample of tears is placed into the reader and the osmolarity is determined by the machine.

InflammaDry

Elevated levels of an enzyme known as *matrix metalloproteinase-9*, or MMP-9, on the ocular surface are considered an indicator of inflammation. When a certain amount of MMP-9 is detected in the tears of dry eye patients, as is a likely finding in connection with dry eye disease, anti-inflammatory therapy may be effective in the treatment of dry eye disease.

InflammaDry is a means of testing for elevated MMP-9 levels. Like a pregnancy test, it does not provide a quantitative result, but rather a yes or no. A technician takes a tear sample from the inside of the lower eyelid with a test strip. After ten minutes, this test strip is analyzed. A solitary blue line indicates a negative result, while a blue line accompanied by a red line indicates a positive result. InflammaDry differs from all other tests for dry eye, which measure tear production or evaporation speed, and can aid in the diagnosis of dry eye in patients whose condition has been missed by other testing methods.

Phenol Red Thread (PRT)

The phenol red thread test is based on Schirmer's test, but instead of a paper strip, it employs a cotton thread that has been treated with phenol red dye, which changes from yellow to red when wetted by tears. The PRT test is used to obtain a quantitative measurement of tear volume. The thread is placed inside the eyelid for fifteen seconds.

Once removed, the portion that changed from yellow to red is measured. Readings of 20 mm or greater are considered normal, while readings of less than 10 mm suggest dry eye. While the accuracy of the PRT test is comparable to that of Schirmer's test, the PRT test takes much less time to administer (a phenol red thread is placed under the eyelid for fifteen seconds, while a Schirmer's test strip must remain under the eyelid for five minutes) and offers little if any discomfort to the patient.

TearScan Diagnostic Tests

Produced by the lacrimal glands, *lactoferrin* is a protein that is present in various secreted fluids, including milk, saliva, nasal discharges, and tears. As such, measuring a patient's lactoferrin level can be an effective way to tell doctors about the adequacy of that patient's aqueous tear production. The TearScan lactoferrin diagnostic test is a noninvasive, quick procedure that allows doctors to differentiate between dry eye due to decreased tear secretion and dry eye due to rapid tear evaporation, as lactoferrin levels are reduced in patients with tear-deficient dry eye.

A doctor collects basal tears from a patient's lower eyelid using a micropipette. These collected tears are then slightly diluted before being placed on a test strip. This TearScan test strip is then analyzed by the TearScan reader. After approximately ninety seconds, the machine will display the amount of lactoferrin contained in the sample. TearScan classifies any result below 0.9 mg/ml as indicative of tear-deficient dry eye. Sometimes doctors use a patient's answers on the Ocular Surface Disease Index to help them decide whether or not to perform this test.

In addition, TearScan also offers a diagnostic test kit for immunoglobulin E, or IgE, a type of antibody associated with allergic reactions. As discussed in Chapter 2, symptoms of allergies can mimic symptoms of dry eye disease. Therefore, it is important to determine the role of allergies when diagnosing dry eye. The TearScan can do so by measuring the IgE level of a patient's tear fluid, which increases along with the severity of a patient's allergic response.

CONCLUSION

As evidenced by the many tests available to diagnose dry eye disease, it may take a number of different investigations into your symptoms in order to acquire an accurate picture of your particular case of dry eye. The results of each test can offer your eye doctor another piece of the puzzle regarding the type of dry eye condition you have, which is crucial information when it comes to determining a treatment plan.

PART TWO

Dry Eye Treatment

A diagnosis of dry eye disease is no cause for panic. While this condition certainly causes discomfort and interferes with your vision, you are not likely at risk of permanent vision loss. You will, no doubt, want to get it under control and hopefully resolved quickly and with as little effort as possible. Part Two starts by listing and explaining the numerous traditional medical treatments that may be employed to combat dry eye, including artificial tears, antibiotics, eyelid scrubs, and other such methods. It follows this information by shedding light on the nutritional approach to dry eye treatment and reviewing the many nutrients that have shown to be effective in the mitigation of dry eye disease. It then lists the most potent food sources of these substances and the supplements you might want to take if your diet is not yet what it should be.

5

*M*edical Treatments

Although it is important to know how dry eye disease develops, how it affects your eyes and vision, and which tests a doctor might use to identify the condition, what you are likely most interested in is knowing how to treat dry eye, whether in a doctor's office or at home. Thankfully, there are many treatment options available to you as a dry eye patient, so therapy can be customized to suit your particular case. While there are a number of dry eye treatments that you can purchase over the counter, most advanced therapies require a prescription from your doctor or need to be administered by your eyecare professional.

AMNIOTIC MEMBRANE

Amniotic membrane is the innermost layer of the *placenta*, which is the structure that provides nutrients and oxygen to (and removes waste products from) a fetus in the womb. The amniotic membrane is the tissue closest to the baby throughout its development in utero. It has anti-inflammatory and antimicrobial properties, which promote a healthy fetal environment.

Like the cornea, amniotic membrane is made up of several layers. The layers of the amniotic membrane include the epithelium, basement membrane, and stroma. The basement membrane consists of different kinds of collagen, including type VII collagen. This type of collagen is also found in the conjunctiva and the cornea. Because many dry eye cases are caused by, or happen in conjunction with, corneal disease, treating the cornea with amniotic membrane is effective in recreating a healthy corneal surface to which the tears can better adhere.

Due to its healing and protective qualities, amniotic membrane is used to help corneal recovery and return the ocular surface to its normal state after eye surgery. It can also treat dry eye by reducing inflammation, keeping the eye moist and protected, and encouraging regeneration of corneal nerves. Its antibacterial properties also help prevent eye infection in dry eye sufferers.

Amniotic membrane is harvested in a sterile environment from placental tissue obtained during elective Cesarean sections. Donors are screened for transmissible diseases before donation, and the membrane is treated with broad-spectrum antibiotics immediately after collection. The membrane is applied (without stitches) over the cornea in a doctor's office, essentially becoming an artificial corneal bandage. It is typically worn for as little as three to five days in mild cases, or for up to fourteen days in severe cases. Lubricating drops are also used in conjunction with this treatment.

ANTIBIOTICS

Dry eye disease has a well-established inflammatory component, oftentimes in connection with an autoimmune condition. Dry eye, however, could also be caused by an infection, especially if there is any involvement with the skin around the eyelids or glands within the eyelids. For the most common forms of dry eye associated with an eyelid infection, a topical (on the skin) antibiotic can work effectively. The form of this antibiotic would be an ointment to be used prior to sleep. If the infection is within the lid or more advanced, an oral antibiotic might be appropriate, but not for pregnant women or women of childbearing age.

ANTI-EVAPORATIVES

When treating evaporative dry eye, obviously preventing the evaporation of the tear film is key. Some products that enhance the lipid layer of the tear film work to reduce evaporation. Unfortunately, most of these types of drops are effective only for about thirty minutes to a few hours, depending on the severity of the dry eye condition. Thus, these superficial treatments, while temporarily soothing, do not address the cause of dry eye or offer any lasting relief.

ARTIFICIAL TEARS

The use of artificial tears is common in the management of dry eye. While artificial tears are typically administered in the form of drops, they can also be applied in the form of a gel or ointment. These supplemental tears dilute the high concentration of salt in the tear film of dry eye sufferers, which can cause damage to the eye. They are meant to lubricate and maintain moisture on the ocular surface, thus alleviating symptoms of dry eye.

As you know, there are several layers to the tear film, so you can imagine how challenging it is to create an artificial tear that can effectively mimic the real thing. Many formulas target one or two layers of the tear film, but rarely all three. New options may offer more customized treatment for patients with severe dry eye symptoms. Like anti-evaporative drops, however, most artificial tear drops provide relief for only a short time.

Different brands have different ingredients, and it may take a few tries to find the right one for your type of dry eye. Some products contain electrolytes, which promote healing of the surface of the eye. Some products contain thickening agents, which allow the artificial tears to stay on the surface of the eye for a longer period. Eye drops with preservatives may have a longer shelf life than those without, but those preservatives can irritate your eyes, which would defeat the purpose of the drops. If you need to use eye drops more than a few times a day, opt for a preservative-free brand.

AUTOLOGOUS SERUM

When a case of dry eye is too severe to respond to artificial tears, *autologous serum* eye drops may be recommended. This serum contains substances artificial tears cannot replicate, including various growth factors and antibodies. Autologous serum encourages nerve regeneration and can heal corneal defects, offering relief to patients who have not found any way to alleviate their dry eye symptoms.

Autologous serum is created from a patient's own blood, which is drawn into a sterile tube and allowed to clot for ten hours. (Patients have approximately thirty vials of blood drawn.) The blood is then centrifuged to extract the serum, which is then diluted to a particular concentration. Bottles of this dilution are frozen for storage. Although this treatment can be expensive, it has been shown to improve corneal health and dry eye symptoms effectively.

BABY SHAMPOO

As you know, one of the primary causes of dry eye is an inflammation of the edges of the eyelids known as blepharitis, which leads to flaking of eyelid skin. This inflammatory condition can affect the functioning of meibomian glands as well as the integrity of the tear film.

To treat blepharitis, some doctors recommend diluting "baby shampoo" with warm water and gently running the solution along the edges of the eyelids with the help of a washcloth. (Use a clean washcloth for each eye.) Due to this shampoo being so mild, it does not cause any irritation to the eye. This treatment, however, has generally been replaced by the use of eyelid scrubs (see page 57), a safe and gentle technology specifically designed to achieve the desired effect.

CORTICOSTEROIDS

Corticosteroids are a type of medicine that has potent anti-inflammatory effects. Proven to reduce swelling, redness, itching, and allergic reactions, corticosteroids are used in the treatment of many inflammatory conditions, including asthma, arthritis, and a number of skin problems.

Concerning dry eye disease, these drugs can reduce inflammation within the tear film, which gives the eye a chance to rebuild the tear film. Doctors typically prescribe the use of a corticosteroid on a short-term basis, and often in combination with the use of artificial tears. Long-term use of corticosteroids can lead to the formation of cataracts. If used for longer than fourteen days, corticosteroid dosage will require gradual tapering under the supervision of a doctor before complete cessation of use.

Eye-Whitening Drops

Many brands of eye-whitening drops claim the ability to "get the red out," but, ironically, most of these drops can produce the opposite result—they can actually make your eyes redder (which will make you want to use more drops to try to get them white again). This redness reappears once the effect of drops, which artificially shrink the size of blood vessels, has worn off, at which point the vessels become even larger than they were before, creating a need to use the eye-whitening drops again. This reaction is called the "rebound effect," and it can lead to a vicious circle of dependence and eventually cause more problems than just red eyes.

Recently, an eye-whitening product called Lumify was approved by the Food and Drug Administration. It claims to lower the risk of the rebound effect by working in a different way to reduce redness. Nevertheless, it contains a preservative that could lead to an unwanted reaction in the eye, so short-term use is favored over long-term use. Ultimately, if you suspect your eye redness might have something to do with dry eye, get your eyes evaluated and treated properly, which should eliminate your desire for eye-whitening drops.

EYELID SCRUBS

As mentioned earlier in this chapter, eyelid scrubs, which are small pads pre-moistened with cleansing solution, have taken over the role of baby shampoo as a means of cleaning inflamed and flaking eyelids due to blepharitis. Perhaps these products should not be called "scrubs," as the edges of the eyelids should never be scrubbed as if one were trying to rub out a spot on a garment. A gentle rubbing action with one of these medicated pads is usually adequate to remove dead skin and clean the edges of the eyelids. Their purpose is to clear the pores located at the edges of the eyelids, which allow lubricating oils to spread onto the tear film.

INTENSE PULSED LIGHT

Intense pulsed light (IPL) is a technology traditionally used by cosmetic and medical practitioners to treat skin conditions such as sun damage, wrinkles, rosacea, and varicose veins. This treatment uses a handheld device to flash intense bursts of light within a certain range of wavelengths on a target area. IPL is being increasingly used in optometry and ophthalmology to treat evaporative dry eye disease due to meibomian gland dysfunction.

To treat meibomian gland dysfunction, intense pulsed light therapy is applied to the lower eyelid near the corner of the eye. The pulsed wavelengths of the light are absorbed by the skin, which reduces inflammation. A special eye shield is worn to prevent the light from hitting the eye directly. This process can be somewhat uncomfortable due to the warmth generated from the light impulses. Most patients experience successful outcomes after three to six treatments spaced four to six weeks apart.

LIPID DROPS

As the name of this entry suggests, these drops increase the thickness of the lipid (front) layer of the tear film. Only one or two drops are required daily, but you may need to use them more often, depending on the cause of your dry eye condition. If your dry eye condition is caused by a lack of tear production, or if the mucin (back) layer of your tear film is not intact, simply enhancing the front layer of your tear film will not be an effective treatment.

EYELID MASSAGE TREATMENT

Eyelid massage treatment removes debris and blockage from the openings of the eyelid glands on the margin of the eyelids. It leaves eyelids and lashes looking much more natural and healthy. It has been shown to relieve dry eye symptoms in affected patients for up to six months. BlephEx is an in-office eyelid massage device that employs a treated micro-sponge attached to a spinning mechanism, while NuLid is an eyelid massage tool that may be used at home. This type of treatment can also be used prior to cataract surgery to decrease the risks of infection and inflammation post-surgery.

NASAL STIMULATION

A relatively new concept in stimulating tear production is the use of a handheld device that is inserted into the nasal canal and electrically stimulates a nerve to produce tears. This stimulation causes an immediate production of mucin by cells in the cornea, oil by meibomian glands, and aqueous fluid by the main lacrimal gland. This unit can be used at home.

There are some concerns with this new technique, which include nasal pain, irritation, and nose bleeds. In addition, it is not intended for those who have a cardiac pacemaker, implanted or wearable defibrillators, or other implanted metallic or electronic devices. The device should not be used for more than thirty minutes in a twenty-four-hour period.

MUCIN SUBSTITUTES

As previously mentioned, the back layer of the tear film is a layer made up mostly of mucous proteins, or mucins. The mucins present in the tear film serve to maintain the wetness of the eye's surface and provide lubrication and anti-adhesive properties between the cells of the cornea and conjunctiva during the act of blinking. They also contribute to the barrier that prevents pathogens from binding to the corneal surface. Therefore, the mucin layer of the cornea is extremely important in maintaining a healthy tear film.

Some lubricating drops act as mucin substitutes. They are specifically formulated to enhance and support the mucin layer of the tear film. These drops can be effective in holding the tear film to the cornea, where the aqueous and lipid layers can build a solid foundation.

OINTMENT

The consistency of most eye drops allows them to flow freely so that they do not distort vision when applied to the surface of the eye. In some cases, however, eye drops dissipate quickly and are effective only for a short period of time. When a long-lasting drop is needed, doctors will often recommend the use of an ointment instead, as this form of treatment has staying power on the eye. Most ointments, however, are thick and tend to distort vision. Therefore, the use of eye ointment is not recommended as a daytime therapy. Rather, it should be applied right before bedtime, when any resultant visual distortions would not pose a problem.

PRESCRIPTION DRUGS

Many of the treatments covered so far are available as over-the-counter products. While this news may sound good to you as a consumer, it may also be a little overwhelming and confusing. Once it had been determined that inflammation was involved in the process of dry eye, pharmaceutical companies set out to develop agents to attack this inflammation with drugs that are compatible with the surface of the eye. For example, Restasis (cyclosporine ophthalmic emulsion 0.05%) was the first pharmaceutical eye drop approved for the treatment of dry eye. This medication treats chronic dry eye disease in connection with inflammation. As an immunosuppressant, this drug suppresses the immune system, preventing it from creating inflammation, which can reduce tear production.

Xiidra (lifitegrast 5%) works by blocking a certain protein on the surface of cells in the cornea. This protein can cause the eyes not to produce enough tears, or to produce tears that are not the consistency required to keep the eyes healthy.

Cequa (cyclosporine A ophthalmic solution 0.09%) increases tear production in patients with dry eye disease. Cequa contains a nanomicellar formulation of cyclosporine, the same active ingredient used in Restasis. Unlike Cequa, however, the cyclosporine present in Restasis is not nanomicellar. The term *nanomicellar* refers to the use of molecules that are one-millionth the size of full-sized molecules of a particular substance. This formulation allows the tear film to absorb a higher concentration of cyclosporine than it would if were treated with a normal formulation of the drug.

PUNCTAL PLUGS

While tears are produced by lacrimal gland and glands within the conjunctiva, they exit the eye through small openings located inside in the edge of the eyelid near the nose. Each upper and lower eyelid has one of these natural drainage valves, known as a *lacrimal puncta*. Once tears exit the eye through the lacrimal puncta, they enter tiny canals known as *lacrimal canals* and drain into a duct called the *nasolacrimal duct*, which is located under the skin and directs the tears into the nasal cavity. This connection between the eye and nose explains why you feel the need to blow your nose after crying.

In the treatment of patients with severe dry eye whose symptoms are exacerbated by excessive tear drainage, punctal plugs may help. Plugging this drainage system, whether temporarily or permanently, can increase tear volume and contact time of natural tears on the ocular surface. Studies show this treatment method can improve patient-reported symptoms of dry eye. This procedure is considered both safe and effective compared with artificial tear use alone, but it is recommended only for patients with drainage system dysfunction. If drainage system dysfunction is not a contributing factor to dry eye, punctual plugs may do more harm than good.

SCLERAL CONTACT LENSES

It might seem counterintuitive to use a contact lens to treat dry eye disease, since many contact lens wearers complain of dry eye symptoms caused by their lenses. There is a particular type of lens, however, that has shown to be effective in reducing the discomfort of dry eye. It is called a *scleral contact lens.*

Most contact lenses are designed to fit predominantly over the cornea, with only the edge of the lens covering the sclera, or white part of the eye. Scleral contact lenses, however, are larger than most traditional soft contact lenses and extend farther onto the sclera. They contain a fluid reservoir into which artificial tears are inserted before the lenses are placed on the eyes. These artificial tears coat the surface of the eye, creating a protective cushion that reduces the pain of inflammation and corneal irritation and alleviates dry eye in the lens wearer.

Scleral contact lenses are recommended for cases of dry eye that have not responded to a more conservative treatment, such as artificial tears, topical drugs, or punctal plugs, and should be considered for use before systemic anti-inflammatory agents or surgery is attempted.

TEA TREE OIL

One of the most elusive causes of dry eye is an infestation of the hair follicles of the eyelashes by the *Demodex* mite. Although this microscopic organism is a normal part of human facial skin, if an overpopulation of *Demodex* mites is not managed, patients may suffer from inflamed and uncomfortable eyelids, leading to dry eye. Once an overpopulation of *Demodex* has been identified, one of the main challenges in treatment is how to kill this tiny organism without injuring the delicate corneal tissue nearby. One of the most effective treatment options is tea tree oil. This oil is derived from the leaves of the tea tree, which is not the same plant that produces leaves for black or green tea. Tea tree oil can kill bacteria and fungus and reduce allergic skin reactions.

Pure tea tree oil, however, is extremely caustic and should therefore never be directly applied to the cornea or conjunctiva. A dilution of the oil is necessary. Patients may wish to use a product such as Cliradex, a natural, preservative-free eyelid, eyelash, and facial cleanser formulated with the most active component of tea tree oil, *terpinen-4-ol*. These wipes can control an overpopulation of *Demodex* mites in eyelash follicles and mitigate symptoms of mite-related dry eye. Cliradex is available as towelettes for moderate to severe ocular irritation, or foam for mild to moderate conditions.

THERMAL PULSATION

Thermal pulse technology uses heat and massage-like pressure to the eyelid to remove gland obstructions and stagnant gland content. An eye doctor or office technician most often performs this procedure. Several devices have been developed for in-office use, and a number of instruments are available for at-home use by patients. Since meibomian gland dysfunction is one of the major causes of dry eye disease, this procedure has become very popular.

One of the most popular thermal pulsate technology units is the LipiFlow. This computer-automated device provides a twelve-minute treatment, during which it heats up and massages the eyelid glands in order to express their contents and reduce retained inflammatory factors. This highly effective treatment is unique, as the heat is applied to the inner eyelid surface directly over the oil-producing gland. It is considered a "high-tech" version of warm compresses. (See the following section.) In affected patients, this thermal pulsation has been shown to reduce dry eye symptoms for up to eighteen months.

WARM COMPRESSES

If your dry eye condition is a result of meibomian gland dysfunction, the oils produced within your eyelid are less fluid than they should be. This oil should have the consistency of olive oil, but as meibomian glands become inflamed, it thickens to a consistency more like toothpaste and is unable to flow easily from its point of origin onto the surface of the eye. As a result, the lipid layer of the tear film begins to thin and lose its integrity, allowing tears to evaporate quickly and the surface of the eye to dry out.

Using a warm compress will soften the oils within the glands and usually allow them to be more easily distributed over the surface of the eye. There are many commercial options when it comes to warm compresses for your eyes, but using a simple washcloth and warm water can allow you to achieve similar results to those offered by these products.

Take a clean washcloth and moisten it with very warm water (warm enough to feel the warmth but not burn your skin). Fold the washcloth and place it over both eyes, applying light pressure for several minutes. After a few minutes, turn the cloth inside out so that it feels warm again. Leave it on your eyelids until it cools. At the end of the process, softly press on the cloth over your closed eyelids. This action will squeeze the glands inside your eyelids and express the softened oils. Using a warm compress several times a day should relieve dry eye symptoms, at least temporarily.

CONCLUSION

Just as there is no one test that can accurately diagnose every case of dry eye, there is no one treatment that will do the trick for every dry eye patient. The good news is that there is an assortment of treatment options out there for this condition. While some of these therapies are available without a prescription and can be self-administered, many require the expertise of your eyecare professional. Any treatment decision should be based on the cause of your dry eye condition, so, even if your symptoms are responding to an over-the-counter therapy, a visit to your eye doctor is always recommended in connection with this problem.

While both prescription and nonprescription medical treatments can be extremely helpful in the alleviation of dry eye disease, taking a nutritional approach to therapy can be a worthwhile endeavor, too, and may even allow you to avoid the need for medical treatment.

Dry eye is typically associated with inflammation, and there are a number of nutrients that fight inflammation and have the potential to reduce symptoms of this troublesome issue—the most common of which are discussed in the following chapter.

6

$\mathcal{T}$he Nutritional Approach

Traditional dry eye treatment typically involves the use of topical medications, often in the form of artificial tears or pharmaceutical solutions used to restore tear production and comfort. Anything other than this approach runs contrary to both conventional treatment protocol and intuition. As science has revealed more about the causes of degenerative diseases, however, we have learned that tear glands are negatively affected by stress and degenerative change just as any other part of the body is. Research has also shown that certain nutrients play a role in mitigating the effects of stress and degenerative change. In fact, studies have demonstrated that specific nutritional components have the ability to restore tear gland function and improve the tear film. To investigate how dry eye sufferers might take a nutritional approach to treatment, we must first focus on essential fatty acids and their connection to free radicals, oxidative stress, and inflammation.

FREE RADICALS, OXIDATIVE STRESS, AND INFLAMMATION

While the electrons that surround the nucleus of an atom always group themselves in pairs, sometimes an electron will become unpaired. An atom or molecule with an unpaired electron is called a *free radical.* Although free radicals are a necessary part of life, they are also highly unstable and reactive. Each free radical is constantly trying to steal an electron from another atom or molecule in order to stabilize itself. As it travels around the body in this attempt, it can cause extensive cellular damage. Once it has stabilized itself, the atom or molecule it used to achieve this goal is left with an unpaired electron and is thus a newly created free radical. This chain reaction will continue until the free radical is neutralized by the body. Age, stress, and degenerative change all appear to be related to a build-up of free radicals in tissue at the cellular level.

The most common type of free radical is the oxygen free radical. Created simply by the act of breathing, oxygen free radicals affect the body on a constant basis. *Oxidative stress* is defined by an imbalance between the production of these free radicals and the body's ability to neutralize them or repair the damage they've caused. Oxidative stress can lead to broken cell membranes, which can alter what enters and exits the affected cells. Eventually, oxidative stress can result in loss of proper tissue function and premature aging of tissue. Just as the stress associated with corneal surgery and contact lens use can lead to dry eye disease, so can oxidative stress. While oxidative stress is one of a number of possible underlying causes of dry eye disease, each of these causes shares a common denominator in inflammation.

Inflammation is the body's way of responding to injury or infection. It signals the immune system to heal damaged tissue or attack unwanted viruses or bacteria. The main symptoms of inflammation include:

- **Pain.** Pain is critical in the inflammatory process, as it lets you know something is wrong. It is the result of inflammatory chemicals that stimulate nerve endings, causing the affected area to feel more sensitive.

- **Heat.** Heat is caused by an increase in blood flow to the affected area.

- **Redness.** Blood vessels of an inflamed area are filled with more blood than usual, so the skin in this area appears red.

- **Swelling.** Swelling is the result of fluid accumulating in tissue. Swelling, however, can occur without inflammation, especially in association with injuries.

- **Loss of function.** Inflammation may cause loss of function, related to swelling of the injured area or illness following the injury.

There are two types of inflammation: acute and chronic. Acute inflammation is a healthy and necessary response that encourages the body to attack bacteria and other foreign substances anywhere in the body. Once the body has healed, inflammation subsides. A chronic inflammatory response, however, may continue to attack healthy areas if it doesn't turn off. It can happen anywhere in the body and may trigger any number of chronic diseases, depending on the area of the body affected. The inflammation that creates a dry eye condition is this type of reaction, which breaks down the immune defenses that reside within the tear film.

There are many established ways to manage inflammation with over-the-counter or prescription medicine, but there is also a nutritional approach that may be taken, the effectiveness of which has begun to be backed up by research. Much of the role of nutrition in addressing dry eye disease has to do with essential fatty acids and their biological effects.

ESSENTIAL FATTY ACIDS

Essential fatty acids, or EFAs, are necessary for life but cannot be produced by the body. These nutrients must be obtained through diet. Available in many foods, essential fatty acids are categorized by length of carbon atoms and the number of double bonds between these atoms. EFAs are typically eaten in short-chain form (typically less than five carbon atoms), but as they are metabolized, various enzymes can cause them to become elongated, leading to the formation of medium-chain (between five and twelve carbon atoms), long-chain (thirteen to twenty-one carbon atoms), or very-long-chain (twenty-two or more carbon atoms) EFAs. Each type of EFA has a role in different actions in the body. Some of them have anti-inflammatory effects, while others can actually promote inflammation, so a nutritional approach to the treatment of dry eye disease would involve lowering or raising levels of certain EFAs in the body.

Omega-6 Fatty Acids

Omega-6 fatty acids are polyunsaturated fatty acids that are crucial to proper brain function, and to growth and development. Due to their ability to halt cellular damage and promote cellular repair, omega-6 fatty acids promote wound healing. They also help regulate metabolism, support bone health, and maintain the reproductive system. While this type of fatty acid is predominantly known to promote an inflammatory response in the body, such as the one associated with wound healing and tissue repair, certain forms of omega-6 fatty acids have anti-inflammatory properties and can lead to the creation of anti-inflammatory substances.

There are several types of omega-6 fatty acids that can have an impact on dry eye disease, including *linoleic acid* (LA), which is the most common dietary omega-6; *arachidonic acid* (AA), which is mainly derived from linoleic acid but may be found in notable amounts in meat and eggs; *gamma-linolenic acid* (GLA), which is also mainly derived from linoleic acid but may be found in borage oil, black currant oil, and evening primrose oil; and *dihomo-gamma-linolenic acid* (DGLA), which is produced from gamma-linolenic acid in an elongation reaction and is the precursor of an anti-inflammatory substance known as *prostaglandin E1.*

Linoleic Acid (LA)

Acquired through the diet, *linoleic acid* is found mostly in vegetable oils, including canola, corn, peanut, safflower, soybean, and sunflower oils, as well as in nuts and seeds. The role of this omega-6 fatty acid in dry eye is minimal in this form. It is only when this short-chain fatty acid is converted into a longer form that it may begin to affect dry eye.

Gamma-Linolenic Acid (GLA)

Although *gamma-linolenic acid* can be found in seed oils such as borage oil, black current oil, and evening primrose oil, dietary intake of this fatty acid is typically negligible. Gamma-linolenic acid is present in the body primarily as a result of linoleic acid metabolism. The conversion of linoleic acid into gamma-linolenic acid can be slowed significantly by stress, alcohol use, smoking, saturated fat intake, or a nutritional deficiency such as a low level of vitamin B_6, magnesium, or zinc. Once GLA has been created, however, it is quickly converted into dihomo-gamma-linolenic acid (DGLA), which is a longer fatty acid than GLA. (See below.) DGLA can then lead to the production of an anti-inflammatory substance known as prostaglandin E1. (See below.) Thus, GLA is an intermediate between LA and the anti-inflammatory prostaglandin E1, although GLA is also able to act directly on the immune system and alleviate inflammation.

Dihomo-Gamma-Linolenic Acid (DGLA)

As recently explained, *dihomo-gamma-linolenic acid* is the elongation product of GLA. Present in only trace amounts in animal products, DGLA is not acquired to any meaningful degree through the diet. DGLA production from GLA is enhanced when high levels of the omega-3 fatty acid alpha-linolenic acid (ALA) are present, blocking the pro-inflammatory pathway. When this happens, DGLA leads to the creation of prostaglandin E1 (PGE1), which is a mucus-specific anti-inflammatory molecule. This substance is especially helpful in resolving dry eye. Like its precursor GLA, DGLA can directly affect the immune system, mitigating the immune system's inflammatory response in connection with autoimmune diseases such as rheumatoid arthritis. Research suggests that treatment with a mixture of LA and GLA can improve the ocular status of patients with Sjögren's syndrome, while this combination has also proven to reduce the expression of the inflammatory marker HLA-DR in conjunctival cells of dry eye patients.

Prostaglandin E1 (PGE1)

While *prostaglandins* are not fatty acids, they are derived from them. They are part of a group of physiologically active chemicals known as *eicosanoids*, which possess hormone-like qualities and produce a wide variety of effects in the body, including encouraging and mitigating inflammation. When a pro-inflammatory prostaglandin is created, it contributes to the development of redness, swelling, and pain at the site of an injury. When an anti-inflammatory prostaglandin is created, it counteracts the effects of the inflammatory process. For example, DGLA yields *prostaglandin E1*, or PGE1, which is anti-inflammatory and powerfully counteracts the inflammatory *prostaglandin E2*, or PGE2, which is a conversion product of the omega-6 fatty acid known as *arachidonic acid*, or AA. Prostaglandin E1 is an anti-inflammatory that stimulates the secretion of mucus, which may benefit the mucin layer of the tear film.

Arachidonic Acid (AA)

Arachidonic acid is an omega-6 fatty acid that is an integral component of the cellular membrane and plays a fundamental role in proper brain and muscle functions. Skeletal muscle has especially large amounts of AA. When cells are activated by particular external stimuli, AA is released from cell membranes and transformed into pro-inflammatory cellular elements. Arachidonic acid can be metabolized by the enzyme *cyclooxygenase-2*, or COX-2, which produces the pro-inflammatory prostaglandin E2. Both *eicosapentaenoic acid*, or EPA, and *docosahexaenoic acid*, or DHA, however, can block the conversion of arachidonic acid into PGE2 by inhibiting the expression of COX-2.

Prostaglandin E2 (PGE2)

Prostaglandin E2 is another example of an eicosanoid. Unlike PGE1, however, this particular eicosanoid is pro-inflammatory substance that is formed when COX-2 metabolizes arachidonic acid. It is a necessary part of the injury response process, causing swelling and pain. While this reaction is important to the healing process, it is unwanted in association with dry eye disease, as it can lead to more dryness and discomfort.

Although you should still include sources of omega-6 fatty acids in your diet, such seeds, nuts, and plant oils, excessive consumption of omega-6 fatty acids can lead to an overabundance of PGE2. The standard American diet already includes far too many omega-6 fatty acids relative to omega-3 fatty acids. Try to achieve a ratio of 4:1, as in four times more omega-6 fatty acids as omega-3 fatty acids in the diet.

Omega-3 Fatty Acids

Omega-3 fatty acids are polyunsaturated fatty acids that play a significant role in normal metabolism. They are important to brain health and are highly concentrated in this organ. In fact, some research has shown intake of omega-3 fatty acids to aid in the recovery from concussions related to high-contact sports. They are crucial to the formation and maintenance of nerve cell membranes, aid in the regulation of blood clotting, balance mood, and ward off cognitive decline. Low levels of omega-3 fatty acids have been associated with poor memory and depression.

Omega-3s also play a necessary part in a number of anti-inflammatory processes and may be beneficial in the treatment of autoimmune diseases such as lupus, eczema, and rheumatoid arthritis. They are widely known to be available in coldwater fish, such as salmon, tuna, and sardines, but are also found in plant sources such as algae, hemp seeds, walnuts, flaxseeds, and Brussels sprouts.

As is the case with the omega-6 fatty acids, there are short-chain, medium-chain, long-chain, and very-long-chain versions of omega-3 fatty acids, and each type is involved in supporting health.

Alpha-Linolenic Acid (ALA)

Alpha-linolenic acid is an omega-3 fatty acid commonly found in seeds, nuts, and vegetable oils. In order to be exhibit significant anti-inflammatory effects, however, this short-chain fatty acid must be converted into a longer form. Thankfully, the body is able to convert alpha-linolenic acid into eicosapentaenoic acid, or EPA, which it then uses to create docosahexaenoic acid, or DHA. These long-chain omega-3 fatty acids are powerful anti-inflammatory substances.

Unfortunately, ALA seems to be metabolized differently by women's bodies than it is by men's bodies. Although both women's and men's bodies convert alpha-linolenic acid into EPA and DHA, research suggests that less than 10 percent of it is converted into physiologically effective levels of EPA and DHA in women, while less than 1 percent is converted into physiologically effective levels of EPA and DHA in men. Thus, men certainly should not depend on ALA alone as a tool to counter inflammation. Both men and women, in fact, should seek out additional kinds of dietary omega-3 fatty acids.

Stearidonic Acid (SDA)

Stearidonic acid is a little discussed long-chain fatty acid that acts as a precursor to longer long-chain fatty acids such as EPA and DHA. SDA is found in such foods as hemp oil, blackcurrant oil, corn gromwell oil, and spirulina, but may also be synthesized in a lab. While ALA has typically been seen as the omega-3 of choice for those who wish to reap the anti-inflammatory benefits of omega-3s without having to eat fish, research suggests that SDA may actually be a better option for vegans and vegetarians to acquire EPA.

Research has shown the conversion of ALA into long-chain fatty acids such as EPA and DHA to be inefficient. It has also shown that SDA metabolism leads to EPA at a rate of three to five times greater than ALA metabolism. Research also suggests, however, that SDA levels do not affect DHA levels, so counting on SDA for all your long-chain omega-3 fatty acid needs is not recommended.

Eicosapentaenoic Acid (EPA)

Eicosapentaenoic acid is one of the most powerful anti-inflammatory fatty acids found in the body. It is found in oily fish, such as cod liver, herring, mackerel, salmon, and sardines, and in various types of algae. In fact, while fish can synthesize EPA from this fatty acid's dietary precursors, much of the EPA in fish comes from the algae they consume. A significant factor in child development, EPA is also found in human breast milk.

The human body converts alpha-linolenic acid into eicosapentaenoic acid. As previously noted, the efficiency of the conversion of ALA to EPA, however, is much lower than the absorption rate of EPA from food. As EPA is also a precursor to DHA and prostaglandin E3, two other potent anti-inflammatory substances, ensuring a sufficient level of EPA in your system, however you accomplish this goal through diet, is very important. It is also important to know that medical conditions such as diabetes or certain allergies can limit the body's ability to convert ALA into EPA.

Docosahexaenoic Acid (DHA)

Docosahexaenoic acid is a long-chain omega-3 fatty acid that is a primary structural component of the human brain, cerebral cortex, skin, and retina. It can be created from ALA or obtained directly from food sources such as breast milk, fish oil, or algae oil. While DHA can be created from the precursor omega-3 fatty acid ALA, the amount of DHA produced by ALA conversion is limited, especially in males.

Docosahexaenoic acid is an even more potent anti-inflammatory than EPA. In addition, cell membranes maintain flexibility and allow nutrients to pass through them more efficiently in the presence of DHA. In terms of the meibomian glands, this nutrient allows them to create oils that flow more efficiently and maintain the integrity of the lipid layer of the tear film.

Prostaglandin E3 (PGE3)

Prostaglandin E3 is an eicosanoid that produces effective anti-inflammatory effects in the body.

EPA and DHA can be converted into prostaglandin E3 by the enzyme *cyclooxygenase*, or COX. This form of prostaglandin can alleviate inflamed tissues and so may be beneficial to the ocular surface.

Bringing It All Together

As you can see from the previous descriptions of essential fatty acids, the nutritional approach to treating dry eye starts with linoleic acid (LA), an omega-6, and alpha-linolenic acid (ALA), an omega-3. Internal enzymes inside the body act upon these fatty acids, producing new substances that have pro- or anti-inflammatory effects. For example, ALA metabolism can produce SDA, EPA, DHA, and prostaglandin E3, all of which have anti-inflammatory properties. LA metabolism can result GLA, DGLA, AA, and prostaglandins E1 and E2. Most of the conversion products encourage inflammation, but a few actually mitigate it.

It must be noted, however, that the enzymes involved in fatty acid metabolism can be affected by many factors. In particular, the level of enzyme *delta-6 desaturase*, which plays a role in both omega-3 and omega-6 metabolism, can be reduced by aging, alcohol, nutritional deficiency, trans fat consumption, and elevated cholesterol. Thus, the conversion of fatty acids may not be as efficient as it appears. As you now understand, simply because omega-6s are predominantly inflammatory and omega-3s are strongly anti-inflammatory does not mean you should shun omega-6s and load up on omega-3s. The body requires a sufficient inflammatory response, so omega-6 are necessary, and even omega-6s can lead to substances that reduce inflammation.

In terms of effectively treating dry eye disease, and of maintaining a healthy body in general, omega-3 and omega-6 fatty acid levels must remain properly balanced to help alleviate this condition. There must be enough ALA to prevent DGLA from taking the inflammatory route and instead encourage it to produce the mucus-specific anti-inflammatory prostaglandin E1. In addition, sufficient amounts of EPA or DHA are needed to block arachidonic acid conversion by the COX-2 enzyme, which results in the pro-inflammatory prostaglandin E2. Of course, sufficient levels of the omega-3s DHA and EPA are also required for the production of the anti-inflammatory prostaglandin E3. PGE3 is an important anti-inflammatory, but it is not as specific to the tear film as prostaglandin E1, which is derived from the omega-6 fatty acid DGLA.

THE RIGHT BALANCE

While the anti-inflammatory effects of omega-3s and omega-6s are of paramount importance when treating dry eye, the overall benefits of the pro-inflammatory properties of fatty acids should not be ignored. Inflammation is necessary to fight infections, diseases, and a host of other conditions. The key aspect of the nutritional approach to treating dry eye is achieving the right balance of essential fatty acids.

The ideal ratio of omega-6s to omega-3s should be about four to one (yes, more omega-6). The standard American diet maintains a ratio closer to twenty-five to one, which means that the pro-inflammatory pathway pushes the body to a state of chronic inflammation. If the proper balance of omega-6s and omega-3s is maintained, however, the omega-3s known as DHA and EPA will block the conversion DGLA into arachidonic acid, which will allow the omega-6 DGLA to convert into the mucus-specific anti-inflammatory prostaglandin

E1. EPA and DHA will also inhibit COX-2 expression and thus the creation of the pro-inflammatory PGE2 from arachidonic acid conversion. These effects will reduce inflammation in all mucous membranes in the body, including those in the tear film.

With the amount of omega-6s so high in the average diet, should we simply increase the amount of omega-3s we take in to reach the desired ratio of four to one? Not necessarily. Given the amount of omega-6s we currently consume, the additional amount of omega-3s required could lead to not-so-beneficial effects. For example, fish oil is a blood thinner, so ingesting excessive amounts to boost omega-3 levels could lead to easy bruising and other blood-thinning effects. A better approach would be to reduce the amount of omega-6 fatty acids in the diet while moderately increasing the omega-3s.

ANTIOXIDANTS

Free radicals are an inevitable part of metabolic processes and relatively harmless as long as they are controlled by the body. When too many free radicals are present, cells and tissues are damaged. Free radicals can cause major damage to the corneal surface and lead to an increase in inflammatory proteins in the tear film, causing dry eye.

We depend on special enzymes manufactured by the body and natural chemicals in our foods called *antioxidants* to neutralize free radicals so that they are unable to do too much harm. Antioxidants commonly derived from food sources include vitamin C, vitamin E, vitamin A (beta-carotene), zinc, and selenium, each of which help defend the body—including the tear film—from harm caused by free radicals. It's important to understand, though, that antioxidants can be easily used up or depleted. Due to this fact, it is important to eat a nutrient-rich diet that provides an abundance of antioxidants and, when diet fails to deliver adequate amounts of these healthful compounds, take supplements that contain these protective substances.

CONCLUSION

Studies have indicated that nutrition can play a substantial role in the health of the tear film and the management of dry eye symptoms.

Research on patients with Sjögren's syndrome has shown that LA and GLA can increase levels of the anti-inflammatory PGE1 and reduce ocular symptoms associated with this condition. Research has also shown that LA and GLA can produce notable improvements in ocular symptoms and ocular surface inflammation in patients with aqueous tear-deficient dry eye. Intake of LA and GLA combined with eyelid hygiene has shown to improve symptoms of evaporative dry eye, which is associated with compromised meibomian gland function, while intake of EPA and DHA has shown to result in significant alleviation of dry eye signs and symptoms.

Not all cases of dry eye will be cured by treatment that takes a nutritional approach, but all dry eye patients will experience some benefit when they add the right nutrients to their diets. Just as you discuss the available medical treatments for dry eye with your doctor, you should also discuss which foods will give your body what it needs to heal itself.

7

*F*oods and Supplements for Dry Eye

N ow that you have an understanding of how nutrients can
support the treatment of dry eye disease, it is time to identify foods that have these nutrients in quantities that can
make a difference. (This book will leave it up to you to incorporate
these foods into your daily meals, but just remember not to add
sugar, which is pro-inflammatory, to dishes in an attempt to make
them more palatable. There are other ways to cook a meal that is both
healthy and tasty.)

Although inflammation plays an important role in the immune
system response and is necessary for survival, chronic inflammation
is stressful on the body and can lead to health problems. Research has
linked dry eye to chronic inflammation, so foods that temper inflammation and thus reduce the symptoms of dry eye are recommended.
The previous chapter explained the anti-inflammatory benefits of
omega-3 and omega-6 fatty acids, and this chapter will list a number
of food sources of these nutrients. Studies have also pointed to free
radicals as a contributor to dry eye. The accumulation of free radicals
in the eye's lacrimal and meibomian glands may be countered by antioxidant-rich foods in the diet.

While it is certainly possible to acquire sufficient anti-inflammatory and antioxidant substances to mitigate symptoms dry eye through

food consumption, the average diet in the United States makes it very difficult to do so. The standard American diet, or SAD, is characterized by high intakes of red meat (typically corn-fed beef), processed meat, pre-packaged foods, butter, fried foods, high-fat dairy products, eggs (from corn-fed chickens), refined grains, potatoes, corn, and high-fructose corn syrup. Instead of fighting inflammation, these foods cause inflammation. Some of these foods may contain antioxidants, but they do not possess nearly the same power to neutralize free radicals as antioxidant-rich fruit and vegetables. Although dry eye sufferers (and everyone else) would be best served by avoiding the standard American diet and incorporating a greater number of anti-inflammatory and antioxidant foods into their diets, there are nutritional supplements that can be used to make up for deficits in these helpful substances. Ultimately, several foods and nutritional supplements have been shown to encourage a healthy ocular surface.

AÇAI BERRIES

Like other berries, the açai (pronounced ah-sigh-EE) berry is packed with valuable anti-inflammatory substances, including *anthocyanins*, proanthocyanidins, protocatechuic acid, procyanidins, and epicatechin. They also contain antioxidant vitamins C and A. In fact, research suggests that the açai berry may have the most antioxidants of any fruit or vegetable, even blue berries and red grapes. It also contains some omega fatty acids. These compounds allow the açai berry to slow down oxidative stress in the body, which is a possible cause of dry eye.

ALOE VERA GEL

Two parts of the aloe vera leaf are used for therapeutic purposes. The gel is found in the inner leaf, while the latex is found just under the skin of the leaf. When the aloe leaf is cut, it is the latex that seeps out. When taking aloe vera internally, use the gel, not the latex, which can cause serious health complications, including kidney failure, exacerbation of intestinal disorders, muscle weakness, and cardiac problems.

The gel of the plant contains fatty acids that give it anti-inflamma-tory, antibacterial, antiviral, and antifungal properties. It also contains pain-relieving substances, hormones that aid in wound healing, and antioxidant vitamins A, C, and E. In fact, there is some evidence that aloe vera gel taken orally may ease the pain of arthritis, a painful con-dition that involves inflammation of the joints.

Aloe vera also encourages mucin cell production and thus sup-ports the mucin layer of the tear film. It is not intended to be applied directly to the eye as an eye drop, however, as it is too thick and would obstruct vision. Instead, it should be taken internally to create the cells that support the tear film. If you drink pure aloe vera juice, keep the amount to about 30 ml (or about one ounce) twice daily. Aloe gel may be mixed into water or added to a smoothie.

While aloe vera latex is the component most associated with dangerous side effects, caution should still be used whenever taking aloe vera gel orally. Begin by taking a very small amount to ensure you are not allergic to the plant. Ingesting any form of aloe is not recommended during pregnancy, as it may cause miscarriage. Aloe should also be avoided during breastfeeding. In addition, diabetics are advised to monitor their blood sugar levels when using aloe, as it may improve the body's ability to control glucose.

Be careful when purchasing aloe vera, as some formulations use the entire leaf, which includes the latex.

BLACK CURRANT SEED OIL

Black currant seed oil contains substantial amounts of omega-6 fatty acids linoleic acid and gamma-linolenic acid, an essential fatty acid found to reduce inflammation specifically in mucous tissue. Gam-ma-linolenic acid can be converted into prostaglandin E1, which pro-duces anti-inflammatory effects. Black currant seed oil also contains the anti-inflammatory omega-3 fatty acid alpha-linolenic acid. Black currant seed oil also exhibits antioxidant properties due to its rich concentration of vitamin C. (The vitamin C content of black currants is estimated to be five times that of oranges.)

Black currant seed oil is generally taken as a supplement. To treat dry eye, take about 800 mg twice a day. Caution should be exercised when using black currant seed oil, as it is known to slow blood clotting. People with bleeding disorders or who take blood thinners should avoid usage altogether.

BORAGE OIL

Also known as borage seed oil, borage oil comes from the seeds of the *Borago officinalis* plant, and has become a popular anti-inflammatory supplement due to its remarkably high concentration of the omega-6 fatty acid gamma-linolenic acid, or GLA. As you now know, GLA is converted into dihomo-gamma-linolenic acid, or DGLA, in the body, which may then be converted into prostaglandin E1, a potent anti-inflammatory. In addition to controlling inflammation, prostaglandin E1 stimulates mucin secretion, which benefits dry eye by supporting the health of the mucin layer of the tear film. Borage oil also has antioxidant properties.

Borage oil is typically taken as a supplement along with evening primrose oil, another source of omega-6 fatty acid GLA, as this combination is known to increase the anti-inflammatory effects of each substance. Moreover, omega-3 fatty acid intake is known to improve results of borage oil supplementation. A typical dosage is about 1.3 g of oil a day.

Results of borage oil supplementation can take weeks to appear. Under no circumstances should pregnant women use borage oil, as it has the potential to induce labor. It can also act as a blood thinner and adversely affect people with seizure disorders, so talk to your doctor before trying this oil.

CHIA SEEDS

It should come as no surprise that the high levels of omega-3 and omega-6 fatty acids in chia seeds can improve dry eye, but what might be confusing is how to eat these seeds. Preparation of these seeds before eating them is highly recommended, as dry chia seeds can expand up to twenty-seven times in weight once added to liquid, which includes the contents of your digestive tract. (In light of this fact, people with swallowing difficulties should avoid chia seeds altogether.) Chia seeds should be soaked in a suitable liquid, such as almond milk or hemp milk, and allowed to expand and soften for at least twelve hours before consumption.

Chia seeds can have a blood-thinning effect, so people on blood-thinning medication should be careful when including them in their diets. They are a good source of calcium, manganese, phosphorus, and other nutrients. A 1-ounce serving of chia seeds contains approximately 49 g of omega-3s and 16 g of omega-6s.

COD LIVER OIL

As its name suggests, cod liver oil is derived from liver of codfish. It contains high levels of vitamin A and vitamin D, which have antioxidant properties, and is a good source of omega-3 fatty acids EPA and DHA. Research suggests that the omega-3 fatty acids and vitamins in cod liver oil can protect against eye diseases caused by inflammation. They can also reduce eye pressure and nerve damage.

Cod liver oil is not used for cooking but mainly used as a supplement, whether in liquid form or as a capsule. There are no set guidelines for liquid cod liver oil intake, but you can safely take 1/2 teaspoon a week, which will boost your EPA, DHA, vitamin A, and Vitamin D levels sufficiently. As vitamin A is fat-soluble and thus tends to build up in the body, higher doses than recently specified are not recommended due to risk of hypervitaminosis A, or excess vitamin A.

Pregnant women should always check with their doctors before taking cod liver oil, as excess vitamin A can harm developing unborn babies. People on blood-thinning medication should also exercise caution when taking cod liver oil, which can act as a blood thinner.

EVENING PRIMROSE OIL

Evening primrose oil comes from the seeds of the evening primrose plant, or *Oenothera biennis*. It is most widely known for its ability to alleviate inflammation. The seeds of evening primrose are abundant in fat, particularly gamma-linolenic acid. GLA's conversion into PGE1 is the main mechanism by which it eases the symptoms of dry eye. In fact, research has show that evening primrose oil can boost levels of anti-inflammatory compounds in natural tears. It has also shown that using evening primrose oil daily for six months can improve dry eye in some contact lens wearers.

As mentioned in the section on borage oil, when evening primrose oil is combined with borage oil, the result is an increase in the anti-inflammatory properties of each substance. Taking between 500 mg and 1 g daily is recommended. It is important to be prudent when taking evening primrose oil, as it may increase the risk of bleeding in people with bleeding disorders or those who are taking blood-thinning medication. People with seizure disorders or who take medication for schizophrenia should also avoid evening primrose oil. Pregnant women should not take this oil either, as it may increase the risk of miscarriage.

FISH

While fish are great sources of the powerful omega-3 fatty acids EPA and DHA, they actually rely on the ALA in algae to make EPA and DHA, just like humans do. In light of the fact that ALA conversion into EPA and DHA is poor, humans may opt to boost their EPA and DHA levels directly by eating fish or taking fish oil supplements. While the following fish are all good sources of omega-3 fatty acids, they also contain many other healthful compounds that not only support the tear film but also overall well-being.

Anchovies

Anchovies are tiny, oily fish. They are typically bought dried or canned and eaten in very small portions. They can be rolled around capers, stuffed in olives, or used as pizza or salad toppings. Their strong taste makes them a distinctive flavor addition to many dishes and sauces, including Worcestershire sauce, remoulade, and Caesar dressing. In addition to omega-3s, anchovies contain notable levels of niacin and selenium. A 3.5-ounce serving of anchovies has approximately 2.1 g of omega-3s.

Caviar

Caviar is essentially salt-cured fish eggs, also known as roe. It is eaten in very small quantities as an appetizer and is considered a luxury edible. Caviar is high in the nutrient choline and low in omega-6 fatty acids. The omega-3 content of 1 tablespoon is approximately 1.1 g.

Herring

Like sardines, herring are rich in long-chain omega-3 fatty acids EPA and DHA, and may therefore reduce a variety of health symptoms related to inflammation, including dry eye. They are also a good source of vitamin D. Another similarity between sardines and herring is that both are close to the bottom of the food chain and therefore do not accumulate contaminants as do large fish. More popular in Europe than in the United States, herring are often salted or pickled, cold-smoked, and then canned for sale. A 3.5-ounce raw Atlantic herring fillet contains approximately 1.7 g of omega-3s. It is also a good source of vitamin C, phosphorus, zinc, magnesium, and B vitamins. It is particularly high in vitamin B_{12}.

Mackerel

Related to tuna, mackerel are high-fat fish that have significant levels of long-chain omega-3 fatty acids. In fact, according to the United States Department of Agriculture, mackerel is close to the top of the list of fish when it comes to omega-3 content, but it is also extremely rich in other nutrients. Like tuna, mackerel has notable amounts of protein and B vitamins, particularly vitamin B_{12}. It is also high in selenium, which has a protective effect against free radicals.

There are several different species of mackerel, the most common of which are king mackerel, Spanish mackerel, and Atlantic mackerel. While king mackerel and Spanish mackerel tend to be high in mercury, the Atlantic species is not, and so is the recommended choice for consumption. While mackerel may be bought fresh, most people purchase canned mackerel. This fish is suitable to be eaten cold or warm, and is so delicious that it needs little to no preparation. A 3.5-ounce serving of salted mackerel provides approximately 2.6 g of omega-3 fatty acids and over 800 percent of the recommended daily amount of vitamin B_{12}.

Oysters

Oysters are an incredibly abundant source of zinc, which works to protect the eye by helping vitamin A create melanin, a beneficial pigment. Zinc deficiency can actually lead to poor night vision or cataracts. Oysters are also rich in iron, copper, manganese, selenium, vitamin B_{12}, vitamin C, and vitamin E. Many of the nutrients found in oysters have anti-inflammatory and antioxidant properties. Apart from fish, oysters are one of the best marine sources of omega-3 fatty acids. Just 3.5 ounces of oysters (six to seven oysters) provide an omega-3 content of approximately 672 mg. Oysters are served raw and can be enjoyed as an appetizer or a whole meal.

Salmon

Although many fish are great sources of the powerful omega-3 fatty acids DHA and EPA, salmon is perhaps the top choice to add to your diet, as it is one of the most nutrient-rich foods you could eat. It is packed not only with EPA and DHA, but also magnesium, potassium, selenium, and B vitamins. The omega-3 content of 3.5 ounces of cooked farmed Atlantic salmon is approximately 2.2g, and wild-caught salmon, which feed on natural sources of algae, have been shown to be an even better source of omega-3 fatty acids.

Sardines

Commonly eaten as an appetizer or snack, sardines are very small, highly nutritious, oil-rich fish.

Like all cold-water fish, they are packed with anti-inflammatory omega-3 fatty acids, which not only mitigate symptoms of dry eye but also help reduce the risks of age-related macular degeneration and diabetic retinopathy, both of which can lead to vision loss. Sardines also contain high levels of many other important nutrients, including protein, vitamin B_{12}, vitamin D, phosphorus, calcium, and selenium, which is also a potent antioxidant. The omega-3 content of 3.5 ounces of canned Atlantic sardines is approximately 1.5 g.

FISH OIL

Although many people confuse fish oil with cod liver oil, these products are not the same. They both come from fish and contain the omega-3 fatty acids EPA and DHA, but fish oil has slightly higher levels of EPA and DHA, and significantly lower levels of vitamins A and D. Like cod liver oil, fish oil supplements can help you get sufficient amounts of EPA and DHA if you don't eat one or two servings of fish each week. EPA and DHA make up about 20 to 30 percent of the fatty acids in regular fish oil, but the fatty acids in highly concentrated fish oils can contain anywhere from 60 to 85 percent EPA and DHA. The anti-inflammatory properties of fish oil can mitigate symptoms of inflammatory diseases and may be beneficial as part of a nutritional approach against dry eye.

Omega-3 fatty acids are prone to oxidation, which makes them go rancid. When choosing a fish oil supplement, opt for one with an antioxidant, such as vitamin E, which will help prevent oxidation. In addition, store the fish oil supplements away from light. Putting them in the refrigerator is a good option. Never take a fish oil supplement if it smells rancid.

Finally, because other fats aid in absorption of omega-3 fatty acids, it is a good idea to take your omega-3s with a meal that contains fat. While the United States has no recommended daily requirement for the EPA and DHA found in fish oil, most studies looking at fish oil's effectiveness suggest a minimum of 1,000 mg a day of EPA/DHA combined. The actual amount of each of these fatty acids can be found on the back of a product's bottle, and adding these numbers together will give you the amount of active ingredient in each capsule.

FLAXSEED AND FLAXSEED OIL

Derived from the flax plant, flaxseeds, also known as linseeds, have a nutty flavor and are often ground and sold as milled flaxseed, flaxseed flour, or flaxseed meal. Ground flaxseed can be baked into any number of baked goods; mixed into smoothies, yogurt, or oatmeal; or sprinkled over salads or sandwiches. Flaxseeds are also used to make flaxseed oil. In terms of experiencing the health benefits of flaxseed, consumption of whole flaxseeds is not recommended, as they are not broken down by the digestive tract, leaving their nutrients unabsorbed by the body. If you buy whole flaxseeds, you would simply have to grind them into powder before eating them in order for your body to absorb the essential fatty acids and other nutrients they contain.

Flaxseeds are an extremely rich source of the omega-3 fatty acid alpha-linolenic acid, or ALA. Moreover, they have a good omega-6 to omega-3 ratio (approximately 1:4) compared with many other seeds. They also contain considerable amounts of *fiber*, magnesium, and vitamin E, an antioxidant.

A short-chain fatty acid, ALA can be converted into the anti-inflammatory long-chain fatty acids EPA and DHA with the help of different enzymes during digestion. This elongation process is hindered, however, by factors such as alcohol consumption, aging, nutrient deficiencies, and elevated cholesterol. It is also affected by gender, with males converting approximately 1 percent of ALA, and females converting about 10 percent. If your main dietary omega fatty acid is ALA, keep these limitations in mind and adjust your intake accordingly. For these reasons, high intakes of flaxseed of about 5 g a day are suggested for women. Given the research that suggests an association between excess flaxseed oil intake and urinary or prostate issues, flaxseed oil is not recommended for men.

Some people take flaxseed oil instead of ground flaxseed. When purchasing flaxseed oil, look for a cold-pressed variety and keep it refrigerated. It is important to note that the oil oxidizes rapidly and becomes rancid, with an unpleasant odor, unless refrigerated. The nutritional value of flaxseed oil is easily destroyed by light as well. Even when kept under optimal conditions, it still has a shelf life of only a few weeks. To avoid the disadvantages of bottled flaxseed oil, many people opt for flaxseed oil supplements, which come in capsule form. This is a convenient choice, although you should speak to your eye doctor to determine how many capsules you should take on a daily basis to treat dry eye.

GRAPESEED OIL AND GRAPESEED EXTRACT

Grapeseed oil is extracted from the seeds of grapes, which are a natural byproduct of wine production. It is high in linoleic acid and has been shown to reduce inflammation. Its significant vitamin E content lends it antioxidant properties as well. While grapeseed oil has a high smoke point, it is not a good choice for high-heat cooking, as its high levels of polyunsaturated fatty acids tend to react with oxygen at high heat and form unhealthy compounds. Grapeseed oil may instead be used in salad dressing, homemade mayonnaise, and baked goods.

There is a concern that grapeseed oil may contain harmful amounts of toxic solvents, which are used during the process of oil extraction. While the vast majority of these solvents are removed during the manufacturing process of grapeseed oil, whether any trace amounts might lead to health complications over time is unknown. If possible, look for grapeseed oil that has been made without toxic solvents.

Grapeseed extract is manufactured using distillation, which avoids toxic solvents, and may be taken as a supplement. While grapeseed oil contains only vitamin E, grapeseed extract, due to its manufacturing process of distillation, contains vitamin E, vitamin A, and vitamin C. It also comprises other antioxidant and anti-inflammatory substances such as flavonoids and polyphenols. Studies have associated a high intake of foods containing omega-6 fatty acids with an increased risk of chronic disease. Controlled studies, however, show that linoleic acid—the type of omega-6 fatty acid in grapeseed oil—does not increase blood levels of inflammatory proteins. A supplement of 100 mg is recommended for daily use.

GREEN TEA AND GREEN TEA EXTRACT

Green tea comes from the leaves of a plant called *Camellia sinensis.* Unlike black tea, green tea is not fermented, allowing it to keep very high levels of antioxidants called *flavonoids,* which provide numerous health benefits, including antioxidant effects. A particular flavonoid in green tea known as *epigallocatechin gallate,* or EGCG, has a high rate of absorption by eye tissues and may improve eye health and fight dry eye. In addition to having antioxidant and anti-inflammatory qualities, ECGC has displayed the ability to protect *retinal ganglion cells,* which are neurons near the inner surface of the retina that aid in the transmission of visual information from the retina to certain regions of the brain. Other antioxidants found in green tea that play a role in vision health include *zeaxanthin* and *lutein.* Studies undertaken in Japan have shown positive physical effects in connection with six cups of tea a day—but this seems to be the norm in Japan. For those people who do not enjoy the taste of green tea, green tea extract is available in capsule form.

Green tea extract may also be used in topical form, which research suggests may be an effective treatment for dry eye associated with malfunctioning meibomian glands. Daily use of topical green tea extract seems to improve the health of these glands and reduce dry eye symptoms without any side effects.

Mucin Enhancers

A deficiency in mucin production can affect corneal health and therefore tear health. Sources of ocular mucin include the conjunctival goblet cells, corneal epithelial cells, and the lacrimal glands. In addition, ocular surface wound-healing growth factors may stimulate mucin secretion by the goblet cells. Mucins produced on the ocular surface have vital functions in protecting vision and preventing dry eye disease.

As mentioned at the outset of this chapter, aloe vera oil encourages mucin prodcution. Other substances that promote mucin production include amino acids such as threonine, serine, proline, and cysteine, which can be found in foods such as soy, meat, eggs, sesame seeds, lima beans, lentils, garlic, onions, and other vegetables. These substances often require other nutrients to be effective, which is yet another reason to eat a healthful diet.

HEMP SEED AND HEMP SEED OIL

Hemp seed comes from the *Cannabis sativa* plant, also called the hemp plant. This plant is widely considered the first cultivated crop by humans, appearing in out earliest written texts. Although *Cannabis sativa* is a source of the drug marijuana, hemp does not possess the psychoactive qualities of this drug, which are the result of the psychoactive component known as *tetrahydrocannabinol,* or THC. Hemp has lower concentrations of THC (less than 0.3 percent) and higher concentrations of *cannabidiol,* or CBD, which can temper the psychoactive effect of THC.

Hemp seeds are an excellent source of nutrition, with a 100-gram serving of hulled hemp seeds supplying 586 calories and 64 percent of the U.S. Food & Drug Administration's recommended Daily Value for protein, making it a wonderful dietary choice for people who would like to cut down or eliminate meat from their diets. Almost half the nutritional make-up of the hemp seed is fat—mainly linoleic acid (55.2 percent), alpha-linolenic acid (20 percent), and oleic acid (10.5 percent)—and approximately 73 percent of its energy content comes from fat.

Hemp seeds are also a rich source of a wide variety of nutrients, including B vitamins, manganese, phosphorus, magnesium, zinc, and iron. They also contain significant dietary fiber and are considered to be less allergenic than other seeds. Hemp seeds can be eaten raw or toasted as a snack. They can also be ground into a fine powder and mixed into a smoothie, sprinkled over salads or cereal, or used as breadcrumbs to coat chicken or fish. Finally, hemp seeds can be blended with water to make hemp milk. Adding 1 to 2 tablespoons to your daily diet may have a beneficial effect on dry eye.

Not be confused with hash oil, which is made from the *Cannabis* flower and contains THC, unrefined hemp seed oil has a nutty flavor and is light to dark green in color. While refined hemp seed oil has a longer shelf life than the unrefined variety, it lacks the antioxidants and other nutrients found in hemp. Hemp seed oil has a relatively low smoke point, which means it starts to burn and release smoke at a low temperature, and thus is not suitable for frying food. It may, however, be drizzled on rice or grains, used as a dip for bread, blended into sauces, or employed as an ingredient in non-sweet salad dressing. (Its strong taste might overpower delicate or sweet dressing.)

A little over three-quarters of hemp seed oil consists of omega fatty acids. These fatty acids occur in a beneficial ratio of omega-6s to omega-3s (approximately 4:1). One tablespoon provides the daily requirement for essential fatty acids. Hemp seed oil supplements are available for those people who do not like the taste of hemp seeds or hemp seed oil.

PINE NUTS

Despite their name, pine nuts are not technically nuts at all. They are the seeds of pine trees. They do, however, possess many of the same healthful nutrients found in nuts, including omega fatty acids and the powerful antioxidant vitamin E. Like actual nuts, pine nuts can become rancid quickly due to their high oil content and should be refrigerated as a preventative measure against this outcome.

A 1-cup serving of pine nuts contains approximately 151 mg of omega-3 fatty acids and 45.4 g of omega-6 fatty acids.

PUMPKIN SEED AND PUMPKIN SEED OIL

Commonly roasted and eaten as a snack, pumpkin seeds are a potent source of many healthful substances. They are packed with magnesium, potassium, calcium, omega fatty acids, and antioxidants such as vitamin E and squalene. The recommended daily intake for pumpkin seeds for adults is 100 g, so about a handful of seeds should be fine.

Pumpkin seed oil contains a variety of fatty acids and is rich in oleic acid and linoleic acid in particular. This oil is also known for its high content of vitamin E and other antioxidants, but only when it is unrefined. Refining pumpkin seed oil reduces its antioxidant content significantly. Pumpkin seed oil is used in salad dressings and marinades, and can even be drizzled over ice cream or fried bananas to give these desserts a nutty taste. Due to its low smoke point, pumpkin seed oil is not recommended as cooking oil.

Like many other healthful oils, pumpkin seed oil can be taken as a supplement in capsule form.

SOYBEANS

Soybeans have received considerable attention in recent years for the many positive effects they can have on health, especially their heart-protective ability. They are a great source of fiber, protein, vitamin B_2, folate, vitamin K, magnesium, and potassium. Their high omega-6 and omega-3 levels can fight inflammation and mitigate the symptoms of dry eye, as can their high levels of antioxidants known as *isoflavones,* which can neutralize the free radicals that might lead to inflammation. A 1-cup serving of cooked soybeans provides approximately 637 mg of omega-3 fatty acids and 4.8 g of omega-6 fatty acids.

SUNFLOWER SEED AND SUNFLOWER OIL

Sunflower seeds are a wonderful source of antioxidant vitamin E. They also provide notable levels of omega fatty acids, especially the omega-6 fatty acid linoleic acid. Sunflower seeds are sold in shelled and unshelled varieties. Their high-fat content makes them prone to becoming rancid quickly, so be sure to buy the freshest seeds you can find. Avoid purchasing unshelled seeds with broken or dirty shells. Shelled seeds that appear yellowish in color should also be avoided, as this color suggests they have probably gone rancid. Store these seeds in an airtight container in the refrigerator. Sunflower seeds can be added to salads, scrambled eggs, cereal, and other meals, or enjoyed on their own as a snack. Consuming a handful of seeds daily may provide dry eye benefits.

Sunflower oil is derived from sunflower seeds and contains significant amounts of vitamin E, vitamin K, *carotenoids,* and selenium. It is also known for its fatty acid content, which consists mainly of linoleic acid and oleic acid. While refined sunflower oil has a high smoke point, which makes it appropriate for cooking, it also lacks the healthful nutrients of unrefined sunflower. Regardless of its smoke point, refined sunflower oil is not recommended. Unrefined sunflower oil should not be used for frying foods either, but may be used in salad dressings, marinades, and dips.

WALNUTS

Walnuts are the only tree nut that contains a considerable amount of alpha-linolenic acid. In every 1/4 cup of walnuts, there are approximately 2.6 g of ALA. Walnuts are also very nutritious in other ways, being a great source of copper, manganese, magnesium, phosphorus, vitamin E, and vitamins B_1, B_6, and B_9. Studies have shown that nuts have remarkable antioxidant strength, particularly walnuts. The waxy outermost layer of a shelled walnut, known as the skin, contains up to 90 percent of its antioxidants, so do not remove this part when eating walnuts. It is one of the healthiest components of the nut.

The Caffeine Question

If you suffer from dry eye, you are likely willing to try almost anything to help ease your condition. You may even want to pick up a coffee habit after reading a couple of small studies that suggest caffeine may increase the amount of tears in the eyes.

One study divided seventy-eight people into two groups, with one group receiving 200 to 600 mg of caffeine in capsule form (about the same amount found in two to six cups of coffee) and the other getting a placebo. It found that the caffeine group ended up having more tears. A smaller study showed a similar boost in tear production from caffeine. This research seems to agree with earlier studies that associate caffeine users with lower rates of dry eye than those experienced by non-caffeine users.

Grabbing a cup of coffee to ward off dry eyes, however, may not be the answer, as there is evidence that caffeine could make dry eye symptoms worse. High caffeine consumption can cause sudden fluctuations in blood sugar levels, which can lead to blurred vision and involuntary twitching of the eyelids. High caffeine intake over a short period of time has actually shown to reduce tear production, causing dry eye.

In addition to having this type of short-term impact on vision, caffeine use over the long-term has been linked to an increase in risk of developing the degenerative eye disease known as *glaucoma*, with a habit of three or more cups a day being connected with this outcome. Caffeine can also lead to an increase in eye pressure, which current glaucoma patients would want to avoid.

VITAMIN A

Vitamin A is the nutrient most commonly associated with eye health. Since the molecule in the retina that converts light energy into nerve energy is a form of vitamin A, this fact is not surprising. Vitamin A is also involved in immune function, reproduction, cellular communication, as well as vision. It also supports cell growth, playing a critical role in the normal formation and maintenance of the heart, lungs, kidneys, and other organs.

In terms of eye health, vitamin A plays supports the integrity of epithelial cells, which make up the front layer of the cornea. Without epithelial cell integrity, the mucin layer would not adhere properly to the cornea, leading to the evaporative form on dry eye.

Sources of vitamin A include orange and yellow vegetables and fruits, broccoli, spinach, and dark leafy greens, which contain the vitamin A precursor *beta-carotene*, which the body converts into active vitamin A. Eggs and meat also contain vitamin A, but in its converted form, known as *retinol* . If you plan on taking a vitamin A supplement, be sure to take note of the form of this nutrient. Vitamin A as beta-carotene does not pose a threat of taking too much, as the body will convert only what it requires, while vitamin A as retinol can lead to serious problems when taken in large doses. Some supplements contain one form or the other, and some include a mix of both. The daily recommended amount of vitamin A is between 700 and 900 mcg.

VITAMIN B$_6$

Also known as pyroxidine, vitamin B$_6$ is a commonly taken as a supplement. It plays a role in the proper digestion of other nutrients, transmission of nerve impulses, creation and function of red blood cells, and expression of genes. It generally serves as a cofactor for many reactions in the body. The liver is the site for vitamin B$_6$ metabolism.

Where dry eyes are concerned, vitamin B$_6$ is required to push the metabolic pathway conversion of GLA into DGLA. In addition, vitamin B$_6$ is required to spark the blink reflex—an especially important mechanism to dry eye sufferers. A dose of 20 mg a day of vitamin B$_6$ should be adequate to help with dry eye.

VITAMIN C

Vitamin C is one of the more popular supplements in the general population. It is a water-soluble vitamin, so it rapidly travels through the body and is excreted in the urine, typically within two to three hours. *Absorbyl palmitate,* however, is a fat-soluble form of vitamin C, which the body can retain for a longer period of time. This form of vitamin C facilitates the production of PGE1, which is the mucus-specific prostaglandin.

This form of vitamin C also enhances the concentration of an antibody known as immunoglobulin E, or IgE, in tears. IgE is the first line of defense against invading pathogens and allergens that frequently cause dry eye symptoms. Taking about 1,000 mg a day in evenly divided doses should assist in easing dry eye symptoms.

VITAMIN D

Vitamin D can improve tear salt concentration and has been shown to work in tandem with vitamin A to ensure proper gene function. Too much vitamin A, however, can interfere with vitamin D's role as an anti-inflammatory in the body, so be sure to keep an eye on the dosage of each vitamin in your supplement regimen. Taking about 150 to 160 IU of vitamin D daily is adequate to balance vitamin A.

Research on tear film function in patients with vitamin D deficiency has shown that people with low vitamin D score significantly higher on the OSDI questionnaire than those who are not deficient in this vitamin, suggesting a connection between dry eye and a lack of vitamin D.

VITAMIN E

Vitamin E is a fat-soluble vitamin that includes four compounds known as *tocopherols* and four compounds known as *tocotrienols.* The most common form of vitamin E available as a supplement is the *alpha-tocopherol* form, which exhibits excellent antioxidant function in the membranes of cells. The addition of vitamin E is particularly important for dry eye treatment supplements that include flaxseed oil or any type of fish oil. Most fish oils and all flax seed oils are easily oxidized and will therefore go rancid quickly if not kept at cool temperatures and preserved with vitamin E, whose antioxidant properties work against oxidation and maintain the freshness of these oils.

LACTOFERRIN

Lactoferrin is a protein found in tears, saliva, and mucosal secretions. It has proven to play a role in supporting and adapting the immune system. In particular, it has demonstrated extremely strong activity against many forms of bacteria. White blood cells stimulate lactoferrin production in the aqueous layer of the tear film, endowing tears with the ability to deal with unwanted invasions by foreign cells.

Adequate levels of tear lactoferrin, naturally produced by the lacrimal gland and white blood cells, are particularly important for eye surgery and contact lens patients, who are disposed to a risk of infection. Lactoferrin supplements are available in capsule form. At least 20 mg a day is adequate for a beneficial effect.

MAGNESIUM

Magnesium may be found in a number of foods, including almonds, avocados, spinach, pumpkin seeds, and tofu. It plays an important role in the transport of calcium and potassium across cell membranes, and as such is crucial to nerve impulse conduction, muscle contraction, and normal heart rhythm. In relation to dry eye disease, magnesium aids in the conversion of omega-6 fatty acids into prostaglandin E1, which supports mucous tissue. Although it is found in many food sources, it is also widely available in supplement form. A dose of 40 mg daily should support dry eye resolution.

CONCLUSION

When it comes to treating dry eye disease with food or supplements, it is clear that anti-inflammatory compounds and antioxidants are the key to success. Omega fatty acids are the main anti-inflammatory nutrients that have proven effective against the condition of dry eye, while a number of vitamins and other substances can provide the anti-oxidants necessary to slow down or even stop dry eye symptoms. The ALA content of certain plant foods can be beneficial in dry eye treatment, but the inefficiency of ALA's conversion into EPA and DHA may drive dry eye sufferers to get their anti-inflammatory omega fatty acids from fish or fish oil instead, which are already rich in EPA and DHA. Plant foods such as seeds, nuts, and berries, however, often pack a considerable antioxidant punch in addition to their omega fatty acid levels, which can be extremely helpful against dry eye.

If you cannot seem to get enough of these therapeutic foods into your diet to relieve dry eye, many of their important compounds can be found in supplement form. Always check with your doctor before starting a supplement regimen, as even the most natural of substances can interfere with the effectiveness of certain medications. Even if you are not on any medications, too much of a good thing can quickly lead to a bad outcome, so be sure to be prudent in regard to supplement dosages.

8

---

*P*utting Things in Plain Sight

We tend to take our eyes for granted. We open them in the morning and the world comes into focus—or it doesn't, which is usually the first sign that something may be wrong with the way we see and possibly with the health of our eyes. It can be especially frightening if our eyes are essentially stuck shut in the morning and cannot open, which is a possibility with dry eyes.

Many healthcare professionals, and indeed even some eyecare professionals, don't feel that dry eye is such a big deal. They might have a point, in that it rarely, if ever, results in a catastrophic, permanent loss of vision. If you are living with dry eye, however, it can wreak havoc on your daily life.

To give you the tools to address this issue, this book begins by covering the basic anatomy and functioning of the eyes and visual system. Recall that the eyes are just the receivers of light and that most of vision occurs in the brain. We tend to think that the first structure of the eye that light hits is the cornea. In fact, it's really the tear film covering the cornea that begins the focusing process of light towards the retina. If this film is not uniform and evenly distributed over the cornea, then vision can be distorted. You will be aware of this if you find yourself having to blink a few times in order to clear your eyesight.

Our tears are made up of three layers: a mucous layer, which holds the tears to the eyeball; a watery layer, which contains a whole host of nutrients and proteins to support the health of the cornea; and finally a fatty layer, which prevents the watery layer from evaporating too quickly. If there is a breakdown in any of these three layers, the eye will not receive the necessary protection normally provided by the tears.

The process of the breakdown of the tear film is still not one that is fully understood by the medical community. The typical scenario goes something like this: The tear film becomes destabilized, which causes a loss of the protection of the inner layers of the tear film. This loss, in turn, causes a drying of the cornea and allows injurious agents into the tear film. These agents include free radicals, toxins, microbes, and allergens, which all lead to inflammation. This inflammation affects the front layers of the cornea, lacrimal glands, and eyelids.

Doctors often begin to check for dry eye by simply asking patients if they feel their eyes are dry at times. Statistics show, however, that a patient's symptoms and the signs of dry eye that can be verified by a doctor don't correlate in about half of cases. In other words, a patient could complain of dry eye but a doctor may not see any objective signs and so would not be able to confirm a dry eye diagnosis. Alternately, a patient may not have any complaints of dry eye but a doctor's tests could reveal a dry eye condition. In light of this problem, there are a number of different tests that doctors must run to confirm a diagnosis of dry eye. In addition, dry eye can be associated with other eye conditions—most commonly allergies.

The most conventional treatment for dry eye disease is artificial tears. (But don't forget that clever marketing has led to people using drops that "get the red out," which can actually make the redness in your eyes worse, causing you to use more drops in an attempt to get your eyes white again. Just having white eyes does not mean they are not still dry!) In recent years, drug companies have developed prescription medications that can increase the production of tears. Some of these can be toxic if taken in large doses, but they can also be very effective. There are a few different classes of this type of medication on the market presently and at least a dozen more in the pipeline.

There is also a significant body of research to support a nutritional approach to treating this condition. The most common nutrients rec-ommended by eye doctors are omega-3 fatty acids, which are abundant in fish oil and certain plant sources. Unfortunately, omega-3s are only one part of the proper nutritional treatment for dry eye. There are several *vitamins, minerals,* other essential fatty acids, and extracts that support the resolution of dry eye and promote eye health in general. These helpful substances include vitamins A, C, D, E, and B$_6$; minerals such as magnesium; and proteins such as lactoferrin.

While the eye is just one of many organs in the body, it is unique in that it allows images from your outer world to enter your brain and be processed. Your eyes provide you with a window to the world, you might say. As they are constantly exposed to the environment, they need to be durable but also moist in order to maintain a clear image. Having dry eyes is not the worst thing that can happen to your vision, but it can certainly interfere with your enjoyment of daily life. By paying attention to your symptoms, sharing this information with your eyecare provider, and following an antioxidant-rich anti-inflammatory diet that supports good overall health, you can alleviate your dry eye condition and see clearly and comfortably throughout your lifetime.

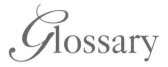

Glossary

This book sometimes uses terms that are common in discussions of eye health but may not be completely familiar to you. You may also hear these terms when working with eyecare specialists. To help you better understand dry eye and its treatment, definitions are provided below for words that are often used by those who diagnose and treat dry eye, and for words that are important in this book. All terms that appear in *italic type* are also defined within the glossary.

absorbyl palmitate. A fat-soluble form of vitamin C, which the body can retain for a longer period of time than water-soluble vitamin C.

age-related macular degeneration (AMD). See *macular degeneration.*

allergic conjunctivitis. A form of *conjunctivitis* that stems from a reaction of the body to an allergen (usually airborne).

alpha-linolenic acid (ALA). An *omega 3 fatty acid* commonly found in seeds, nuts, and vegetable oils. In order to be exhibit effective anti-inflammatory effects, however, this short-chain fatty acid must be converted into a longer form. Thankfully, the body is able to convert it into *eicosapentaenoic acid.*

alpha-tocopherol. The most common form of vitamin E available as a supplement. It exhibits excellent *antioxidant* function in the membranes of cells.

amino acids. The building blocks of *proteins.* There are twenty amino acids. Eleven of them can be made by the body and are considered nonessential because they don't have to be supplied by the diet. The nine amino acids that must be supplied by the diet are considered essential.

amniotic membrane. The innermost layer of the *placenta.*

anthocyanins. Red, blue, and purple pigments that are found in many fruits and vegetables—including the seeds of red grapes—and provide protection against *oxidative stress* and *inflammation.*

antioxidants. Powerful substances that block oxidation by neutralizing substances called *free radicals,* which otherwise can lead to the dysfunction and destruction of cells. The wide range of *antioxidant* nutrients includes *beta-carotene,* vitamin C, vitamin E, and selenium. They are mostly found in fresh fruit and vegetables.

aqueous humor. A clear fluid that fills the small chamber between the *cornea* and the *iris* and provides some nutrition to the adjoining parts of the eye. It flows in and out of the eye on a regular basis.

aqueous layer. The thickest portion of the *tear film.* As its name suggests, it is the watery component of the *tear film.* It hydrates the *cornea,* flushes out particles, and helps prevent infection. It also contains many of the nutrients that support the health of the *cornea.*

aqueous tear-deficient dry eye. A type of dry eye disease associated with dysfunction in the tear glands. This dysfunction makes the tear glands unable to produce a sufficient amount of tears.

arachidonic acid (AA). An *omega-6 fatty acid* mainly derived from *linoleic acid,* but which may be found in notable amounts in meat and eggs.

autoimmune disease. A condition in which the immune system malfunctions, attacking normal cells in the body.

autologous serum. A serum that contains substances artificial tears cannot replicate, including various growth factors and antibodies.

basal tears. Tears produced by glands in the *conjunctiva.* They lubricate the eye and help to keep it clear of dust and debris.

beta-carotene. A *carotenoid* that is converted by the body into active vitamin A. Beta-carotene is an excellent *antioxidant* that may help protect the *macula* against *oxidative stress.*

blepharitis. Swollen eyelids due to *inflammation* of the *meibomian glands.*

blood glucose. See *blood sugar.*

blood sugar. The main sugar found in the blood.

carotenoids. Plant-derived pigments that give plants their bright yellow, orange, and red colors and act as strong *antioxidants* to reduce *oxidative stress.* There are over sixty carotenoids found in foods, the most famous of which is *beta-carotene.*

cataract. A clouding of the lens of the eye.

choroid. The middle layer of the eye wall sandwiched between the *sclera* and the *retina.* The choroid is filled with blood vessels that deliver oxygen and nutrients to the *retina* and to other structures found inside the eye.

crystalline lens. See *lens.*

cones. The specialized cone-shaped *photoreceptors* embedded in one layer of the *retina.* Because cones are active in high levels of light and respond to colors, they are essential to daytime vision. Our sharpest vision comes from cones.

conjunctiva. The thin, normally transparent membrane that covers the *sclera* and lines the eyelids.

conjunctivitis. *Inflammation* of the *conjunctiva.*

cornea. The transparent dome-shaped structure that covers the front of the eye. It acts as the eye's outermost *lens*, functioning as a window that helps focus the entry of light into the eye.

corticosteroid. A type of medicine that has potent anti-inflammatory effects. Proven to reduce swelling, redness, itching, and allergic reactions, corticosteroids are used in the treatment of many inflammatory conditions, including asthma, arthritis, and a number of skin problems.

cyclooxygenase (COX). An *enzyme* that converts EPA and DHA into *prostaglandin E3*, which can alleviate inflamed tissues and so may be beneficial to the ocular surface.

cytokines. *Proteins* that serve as molecular messengers between cells. Cytokines interact with cells of the immune system, leading to inflammatory or anti-inflammatory responses.

delta-6 desaturase. An *enzyme* that plays a role in both omega-3 and omega-6 metabolism. It can be reduced by aging, alcohol, nutritional deficiency, trans fat consumption, and elevated cholesterol.

Demodex. A genus of tiny mites that live in or near hair follicles of mammals.

diabetes. A condition characterized by an abnormal metabolism of carbohydrates that leads to elevated *blood glucose* levels.

diabetic retinopathy. An eye disease caused by *diabetes* in which blood vessel walls are weakened, causing the small blood vessels inside the eye to become more fragile. The blood vessels then leak fluid and blood into the center of the eye, causing loss of vision.

dihomo-gamma-linolenic acid (DGLA). An omega-6 fatty acid produced from *gamma-linolenic acid* in an elongation reaction. It is the precursor of an anti-inflammatory substance known as *prostaglandin E1*.

docosahexaenoic acid (DHA). A long-chain *omega-3 fatty acid* that is a primary structural component of the human brain, cerebral cortex, skin, and *retina*. It can be created from *ALA* or obtained directly from food sources such as breast milk, fish oil, or algae oil.

dry eye syndrome (DES). One of the original terms used to describe a disorder of the tear film caused by diminished tear production or excessive tear evaporation.

dry eye disease (DED). A term coined by the Tear Film and Ocular Society to describe disorder of the *tear film*. Dry eye disease refers to a multifactorial disease of the ocular surface characterized by a loss of homeostasis (physiological balance) of the *tear film*, and accompanied by ocular symptoms, in which tear film instability and hyperosmolarity, ocular surface *inflammation* and damage, and neurosensory abnormalities play etiological roles.

dysfunctional tear syndrome (DTS). A term coined by a group of international professional researchers known as the Delphi Panel to describe disorders of the *tear film*.

eicosanoids. Substances that possess hormone-like qualities and produce a wide variety of effects in the body, including encouraging and mitigating *inflammation*.

eicosapentaenoic acid (EPA). One of the most powerful anti-inflammatory fatty acids. EPA is found in oily fish, such as cod liver, herring, mackerel, salmon, and sardines, and in various types of algae. The human body can also convert *alpha-linolenic acid* into eicosapentaenoic acid.

enzyme. A type of *protein* that is capable of inducing chemical changes in other substances without being changed itself.

epigallocatechin gallate (EGCG). A *flavonoid* found in green tea. It has a high rate of absorption by eye tissues and may improve eye health and fight dry eye.

epithelial cells. The cells that make up the tissues that line the outer surfaces of organs and blood vessels.

essential fatty acids (EFAs). Special dietary fats that are termed "essential" because they are required for good health but cannot be made by the body, and therefore must be consumed in food or supplements. There are two EFA families: *omega-3 fatty acids* and *omega-6 fatty acids*.

evaporative dry eye. A type of *dry eye disease* associated with an abnormally quick evaporation of tears from the surface of the eye.

exocrine glands. Glands that produce and secrete substances onto a surface of the body.

fiber. A type of carbohydrate, also referred to as roughage, which is found only in plants and cannot be broken down by digestion and absorbed by the body. There are two types of fiber: soluble and insoluble. Soluble fiber dissolves in water, while insoluble fiber does not.

flavonoids. These nutrients add flavor and color to fruits and vegetables and are important in preventing and treating eye disease because of their strong *antioxidant* activity. They convert highly reactive *free radicals* to less reactive free radicals, improve blood flow to the eye, and are anti-inflammatory.

floaters. Substances that are suspended in the *vitreous humor.*

fovea. A small dimple found in the middle of the *macula*, where *visual acuity* is the highest.

free radicals. Atoms or groups of atoms with an odd (unpaired) number of electrons. Once formed, *free radicals* scavenge the body to seek out other electrons to complete the pair. This process causes injury to cells, *proteins*, and DNA.

gamma-linolenic acid (GLA). An *omega-6 fatty acid* mainly derived from *linoleic acid*, but which may be found in borage oil, black current oil, and evening primrose oil.

ganglion cells. Specialized nerve cells that receive signals from the *rod* and *cone photoreceptors.*

glaucoma. A condition marked by abnormally high eye pressure.

goiter. An enlargement of the thyroid gland.

hyperthyroidism. Dysfunction of the thyroid gland defined by an overactive thyroid.

hypothyroidism. Dysfunction of the thyroid gland defined by an underactive thyroid.

immunoglobulin E (IgE). An antibody found in tears. IgE is the first line of defense against invading pathogens and allergens that frequently cause dry eye symptoms.

inflammation. A reaction of the immune system to harmful stimuli that can include swelling, redness, and pain.

insulin. A hormone that allows *glucose,* or sugar, to enter the cells and be used as an energy source.

iris. The ring-shaped colored portion of the eye that surrounds the *pupil* and regulates the amount of light that enters the eye. The iris contains muscles that allow the *pupil* to dilate (open) when there is relatively little light, and constrict (get smaller) when the light is bright.

keratitis. An *inflammation* of the *cornea.*

keratoconjunctivitis sicca (KCS). See *dry eye syndrome.*

keratograph. A device that uses infrared illumination to measure *tear break-up time* noninvasively, without the need to use any dye.

lacrimal canals. Tiny canals into which tears enter upon exiting the *lacrimal puncta,* and through which tears drain into the *nasolacrimal duct.*

lacrimal glands. Glands located in several places around the eye that produce tears.

lacrimal puncta. Natural drainage valves located in the upper and lower eyelids.

lactoferrin. A *protein* present in various secreted fluids, including milk, saliva, nasal discharges, and tears.

lens. Sometimes called the *crystalline lens,* the resilient, transparent structure behind the *iris* that focuses light on the *retina* by changing the curvature of its front surface.

leukocytes. See *white blood cells.*

linoleic acid (LA). The most common dietary *omega-6 fatty acid.*

lipid layer. The outermost portion of the *tear film.* It is produced by the *meibomian glands,* which are located within the structure of the eyelids. This oil-based component coats the *aqueous layer* of the *tear film,* providing a seal, which reduces the evaporation of the tear layers below and limits the spillage of tears onto the cheeks.

lupus. See *systemic lupus erythematosus.*

lutein. A *carotenoid* present in certain foods, especially dark leafy greens like kale and spinach. Lutein is present in high concentrations in the *macula*. A pigment, lutein helps give the macula its yellowish color and guards the eye from the damaging effects of light.

lymphocytes. One of the body's main types of *white blood cells.*

macula. The central area of the *retina* that is used for sharp, detailed vision, such as that needed for reading and sewing. Together with the *fovea*, it forms the *macular region*, which is the region that is affected by *macular degeneration.*

macular degeneration. An eye disorder that progressively destroys the *macula*, the central portion of the *retina* that is needed for central vision. Macular degeneration is the leading cause of vision loss in adults aged fifty and over.

macular region. The region of the eye made up of the *fovea* and the *macula*.

matrix metalloproteinase-9 (MMP-9). An *enzyme* whose presence on the ocular surface is considered an indicator of *inflammation.*

meibomian gland dysfunction (MGD). A condition defined by abnormal *meibomian gland* function, which can cause tears to evaporate too quickly, making it a leading cause of dry eye.

meibomian glands. These glands produce the oils that make up the *lipid layer*, which are squeezed out of these glands and spread over the eye with each blink.

minerals. Naturally occurring substances that are solid and inorganic, meaning that they don't contain carbon. Minerals must be consumed in the diet because the body needs them for important functions but cannot produce them.

mucin layer. The innermost layer of the *tear film*, closest to the *cornea*. Produced predominantly by goblet cells in the *conjunctiva, mucins* are proteins that form a gel-like coating of mucus over the *cornea*. This layer of mucus allows the watery layer above it to wet the surface of the *cornea* evenly, helping it to retain moisture.

mucins. *Proteins* that form a gel-like coating of mucus.

nanomicellar. Referring to the use of molecules that are one-millionth the size of full-sized molecules of a substance.

nasolacrimal duct. A duct located under the skin below the eye. It directs tears into the nasal cavity.

ocular rosacea. Eye complications associated with rosacea, including redness, burning, stinging, and irritation of the eye, and the feeling of a foreign substance in the eye.

ocular surface disease (OSD). A term that is used interchangeably with *dry eye disease.*

omega-3 fatty acids. A special class of *essential fatty acids* that includes *alpha-linolenic acid, EPA,* and *DHA.* Omega-3 fatty acids play a role in maintaining healthy cell membranes and are anti-inflammatory and *antioxidant* in their effects.

omega-6 fatty acids. A special class of *essential fatty acids* that includes linoleic acid. Omega-6 fatty acids have many important functions in the body, but if eaten in excess, can have negative effects such as increased *inflammation* and higher blood pressure.

optic nerve. A nerve that uses electrical impulses to transfer visual information received by the *retina* to the vision centers of the brain.

osmolarity. The saltiness of tears.

oxidative stress. An imbalance between the production of *free radicals* and the ability of the body to neutralize the *free radicals* with *antioxidants.* Oxidative stress is associated with many serious disorders, including heart disease.

pancreatic beta cells. Insulin-producing cells.

photoreceptors. Sensory cells found in the *retina* that are stimulated by light. They include the *cones* and the *rods.*

pink eye. See *conjunctivitis.*

placenta. A structure that provides nutrients and oxygen to (and removes waste products from) a fetus in the womb.

precorneal film. See *tear film.*

prediabetes. A condition in which blood glucose levels are higher than normal, but not high enough for a diagnosis of fully developed *diabetes.*

prostaglandin E1 (PGE1). A mucus-specific anti-inflammatory molecule. This substance is especially helpful in resolving dry eye.

prostaglandin E2 (PGE2). An inflammatory conversion product of the *omega-6 fatty acid* known as *arachidonic acid.*

prostaglandin E3 (PGE3). An *eicosanoid* that produces effective anti-inflammatory effects in the body. *EPA* and *DHA* can be converted into prostaglandin E3 by the enzyme *cyclooxygenase.* This form of *prostaglandin* can alleviate inflamed tissues and so may be beneficial to the ocular surface.

prostaglandins. Derived from fatty acids, these substances are part of a group of physiologically active chemicals known as *eicosanoids,* which possess hormone-like qualities and produce a wide variety of effects in the body, including encouraging and mitigating *inflammation.*

protein. A nutrient made from *amino acids* that is needed in all body cells for the structure, function, and regulation of body tissues and organs.

psychic tears. Tears that occur in response to strong emotions, such as sadness, extreme stress, or even happiness.

pupil. The opening in the center of the *iris* that allows light to enter the eye so it can be focused on the *retina.*

recurrent corneal erosion. A condition defined by the wearing away of corneal cells, typically caused by a trauma or genetic defect.

reflex tears. Tears produced and secreted in response to the presence of an irritant such a foreign body or irritant fumes.

retina. A thin layer of tissue that lines the back of the eye. Its purpose is to receive the light that has been focused by the *lens,* convert it into neural signals, and send these signals to the brain, where they are transformed into an image.

rheumatoid arthritis (RA). An *autoimmune disease* that causes pain, stiffness, swelling, and loss of function in the joints.

rods. The specialized rod-shaped *photoreceptors* embedded in one layer of the *retina*. The rods are responsible for vision in low levels of light, and therefore are essential to night vision.

rosacea. A chronic skin condition of the facial area. It is characterized by symptoms such as facial flushing, skin redness, spider veins, skin coarseness, and inflammatory eruption of the skin similar to acne.

sclera. The dense white outer covering of the eye that is sometimes known as the white of the eye. Its main purpose is to support and protect the inner eye structures and attach the eye to the six muscles that control its movement.

scleral contact lenses. Contact lenses that are larger than most traditional soft contact lenses and extend farther onto the *sclera*. They contain a fluid reservoir into which artificial tears are inserted before the lenses are placed on the eyes.

Schirmer's test. A dry eye examination in which a paper strip is inserted into the space between the eyeball and the lower eyelid for several minutes to measure the production of tears.

Sjögren's syndrome. An *autoimmune disease* in which the immune system attacks the glands that make tears and saliva, leading to dry mouth and *dry eye disease.*

stearidonic acid (SDA). A little discussed long-chain fatty acid that acts as a precursor to longer long-chain fatty acids such as *EPA* and *DHA.* SDA is found in such foods as hemp oil, blackcurrant oil, corn gromwell oil, and spirulina, but may also be synthesized in a lab.

systemic lupus erythematosus (SLE). More commonly known as *lupus,* systemic lupus erythematosus is a chronic *autoimmune disease* that exhibits a wide range of symptoms due to its impact on virtually every organ. Common symptoms of lupus include fever, joint pain, rash, and dry eye.

tear break-up time (TBUT). The number of seconds that elapse between a blink of an eye and the appearance of the first dry spot on this eye.

tear film. A thin film that floats in front of the *cornea*, moisturizing, nourishing, and protecting the eye.

terpinen-4-ol. The most active component of tea tree oil.

visual field. The entire area that can be seen without shifting the position of the eyes. It includes both central and peripheral vision.

vitamins. Organic molecules (meaning that they contain carbon atoms) that must be consumed as part of the diet because they cannot be made by the body.

vitreous humor. A clear gel-like substance that fills the large central chamber of the eye between the *lens* and the *retina*.

white blood cells. Infection-fighting components of the immune system.

zeaxanthin. A *carotenoid* present in certain foods, such as red peppers and carrots. Zeaxanthin is present in high concentrations in the *macula*. A pigment, zeaxanthin guards the eye from the damaging effects of light.

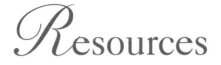

Resources

There are dozens and dozens of options in the treatment of dry eye. This section provides information on a number of at-home treatments and support groups that might be of help to you in your journey towards eye health. This section also includes a list of products that is intended to help you find the right remedies for your particular case of dry eye. This list is by no means complete and the products it contains are subject to change at any time.

SUPPORT GROUPS

Support groups can provide dry eye sufferers with helpful information and encouragement. There are a number of beneficial online dry eye groups and forums, but you may also wish to attend a support group meeting in person. You may find a local support group and its meeting schedule by doing an online search for dry eye support groups in your area.

Daily Strength Dry Eyes Support Group
Daily Strength
Website: www.dailystrength.org/
group/dry-eyes

Dry Eye Syndrome Support Community
Website: www.facebook.com/
groups/dryeyesupport/
?ref=group_header

The Dry Eye Zone Forums
The Dry Eye Zone
Website:
www.forum.dryeyezone.com

Sjögren's World Forums
Sjögren's World
Website:
www.sjogrensworld.org/forums

NUTRITIONAL SUPPLEMENTS

In light of the fact that diet can actually impact the tear film, many companies have developed nutritional supplements to combat dry eye. Omega fatty acids play a big role in the quality of the tear film, so many of these products are based on these nutrients. Omega-3s, however, are only part of the therapeutic picture. Look for a supplement that maintains a complete spectrum of nutrients that support the tear film.

Bio Tears

Biosyntrx
Website: https://biosyntrx.com
Bio Tears combines nutrient cofactors that support the body's natural lubrication of the eyes, including omega-6 fatty acids from black currant seed oil, omega-3 fatty acids from fish oil and pharmaceutical grade cod liver oil, vitamin A, vitamin E, vitamin C, curcumin, lactoferrin, and green tea. These ingredients are designed to work synergistically rather than individually.

Dry Eye Omega Benefits

PRN
Website:
   https://prnomegahealth.com
Dry Eye Omega Benefits is uniquely formulated and patented to provide relief from occasional dry eye. Dry Eye Omega Benefits provides the right quantities of omega-3s EPA and DHA in the right ratio and most easily absorbable form. It is available as a softgel or liquid.

EyeScience Dry Eye Formula

EyeScience
Website: www.eyescience.com
EyeScience Dry Eye Formula softgels are an oral supplement that uses high levels of omega-3s to help improve tear production and seal in moisture for lasting comfort, working from the inside of the eye to the outside and continuously addressing the underlying cause of occasional dry eye.

EyePromise EZ Tears

ZeaVision
Website: www.eyepromise.com
EyePromise EZ Tears is designed to encourage the body to produce more tears with a greater level of lubrication to relieve dry eye discomfort and irritation. It is formulated to work fast and address occasional dry eye in as little as one week, soothing burning, itchy eyes, and allowing people to wear their contact lenses longer and reduce eye drop use.

HydroEye

ScienceBased Health
Website:
   www.sciencebasedhealth.com
HydroEye is a patented nutritional formulation that provides continuous support for dry eyes by delivering a proprietary blend of omega fatty acids (GLA, EPA, and DHA), antioxidants,

and other key nutrients. These ingredients work together to support a healthy tear film and soothe the ocular surface.

Tear Support Plus
Lunovus
Website: https://lunovus.com

Lunovus's Tear Support Plus is a supplement designed to promote the production of tears. The Tear Support Plus softgels are made in an FDA-inspected facility in the United States. The company employs vigorous testing and quality assurance to ensure

their supplements are pharmaceutical grade. The Tear Support Plus formula combines omega-3s, omega-7s, and vitamin D.

TheraTears Eye Nutrition
TheraTears
Website: www.theratears.com

Designed to promote healthy tears, TheraTears Eye Nutrition offers an optimized blend of organic flaxseed oil, a triglyceride form of fish oil, and Vitamin E. It is available in softgel form.

AT-HOME TREATMENTS

There are literally dozens of eyelid masks and treatments on the market. Here are a few of the more popular ones. While the use of a mask may be helpful in the treatment of dry eye, it is not absolutely required for successful resolution of this problem. If you have only enough time to use a mask once a day, do so prior to sleep. You can even make a homemade version by wetting a clean washcloth thoroughly with very warm water, folding it in half, and applying it to your closed eyes for about three minutes. When it starts to cool, turn it inside out and reapply it to your closed eyes for another two minutes. Before removing it for the last time, press down on your closed eyelids gently several times to massage them through the washcloth.

Blephadex Warming Eyelid Wipes
Website: www.blephadex.com

These pre-moistened eyelid wipes are made with tea tree oil and coconut oil. They produce a warming effect, which is stimulated by an innovative water-activated heat technology and softens oils in the meibomian glands, allowing increased flow onto the tear film.

Blink Lid Wipes
Website: www.justblink.com

These pre-moistened eyelid wipes use chamomile as an active ingredient. They are ideal for removing debris and crusting from eyelids and lashes. They are also suitable for contact lens wearers.

Bruder Hygienic Eyelid Solution

Bruder

Website: www.bruder.com

This eyelid spray is to be used on closed eyes to cleanse the eyelid margins. It contains a proprietary form of hypochlorous acid, a natural antibacterial substance, but is free of alcohol, sulfates, parabens, and added fragrance.

Bruder Moist Heat Eye Compress

Bruder

Website: www.bruder.com

The Bruder Moist Heat Eye Compress opens oil glands and allows natural oils to flow back into the eye, relieving discomfort. The compress helps stabilize the tear film, improves oil gland function, and slows tear evaporation. It is washable, reusable, and self-hydrating, which means there is no need to add water.

Cliradex Towelettes

Cliradex

Website: https://cliradex.com

This natural eyelid cleanser includes a powerful component of tea tree oil, which is especially effective against Demodex mites, and is free of parabens, fillers, artificial colors, and alcohol. It is designed to relieve symptoms of dry eye, blepharitis, Demodex, and other eyelid or skin conditions. It is meant to treat symptoms of moderate to severe ocular irritation due to blepharitis, Demodex, or other eyelid conditions.

EyeGiene Insta-Warmth System

EyeGiene

Website: www.eyegiene.com

The EyeGiene Insta-Warmth System is different than most warm compress masks in that is does not require a microwave to heat. This product combines a soft eye mask and disposable warming wafers to deliver precise warm compress treatment to the eyelids. The mask comes with ten disposable warming wafers, and refills may be purchased.

The Eyelid Scrub Kit

We Love Eyes

Website: www.weloveeyes.com

This kit includes cleansing oil and foaming cleanser made from tea tree oil, grapeseed oil, and jojoba oil. It is administered in two steps and delivers relief to patients with meibomian gland disorders, dry eye, and blepharitis. It reduces bacteria, dirt, and allergens that can cause inflammation. It is also safe to use with eyelash extensions.

Flaxseed Dry Eye Warm Compress Mask

Eye Love

Website: www.eyelovethesun.com

The Flaxseed Dry Eye Warm Compress Mask is a more natural option than other masks for those suffering from dry eye. It has no added chemicals and is filled with all-natural ingredients that don't irritate the eyes. It has a silk covering and contains flaxseed and lavender. It may be used as a warm compress or a cold compress, and has silk ties that allow it to fit any head shape.

Heyedrate Dry Eye Mask

Eye Love

Website: www.eyelovethesun.com

The Heyedrate Dry Eye Mask is a great option for those who want advanced technology without the high price. The beads inside the mask absorb water from the air, so after the mask has been heated in the microwave, it produces a moist heat, which maintains its high temperature for a long period of time, leaving your oil glands easier to express. This compress is freezer safe, so you can also use it as a cold compress.

Hypochlor

Ocusoft

Website: www.ocusoft.com

When combined with a product such as Ocusoft Lid Scrub in the removal of oil and debris from the eyelids, Hypochlor can be effective in the treatment of severe cases of eyelid discomfort. It is the strongest cleansing solution available without a prescription.

Manuka Honey Eyelid Cleanser

Honey Clear

Website: https://beehoneyfit.com

This eyelid cleanser contains cosmetic-grade manuka honey, which possesses antibacterial properties. It gently removes bacteria, debris, and other irritants on the eyelids. It is particularly recommended for people with blepharitis, Demodex, or dry eye symptoms.

Mediviz Blepharitis Eye Mask

The Mediviz Blepharitis Eye Mask's MediBeads technology makes it very similar to the Heyedrate Dry Eye Mask, although this mask is a little more expensive than Heyedrate's version. This compress offers a machine-washable cover, which allows the mask to be used hygienically over time. It is available for purchase on many vision-related websites.

Oasis LID & LASH + Tea Tree Oil Cleansing Pads

Oasis

www.oasis.com

These lightly abrasive pads are soaked in a hydrating gel cleanser soaked for daily eyelid and lash hygiene. The gentle cleanser hydrates delicate skin around the eyes and gently removes eye debris and dust particles as it cleanses.

Ocusoft Lid Scrub

Ocusoft

Website: www.ocusoft.com

The pores of the meibomian glands, which empty oils onto the eyelid margins, must be clear and free from debris (dead skin cells, etc.) This non-irritating formula effectively removes oil, debris, and pollen from the eyelids. It is ideal for daily eyelid hygiene, and to treat mild to moderate eyelid conditions, which can lead to dry eye.

Ocusoft Lid Scrub Plus Platinum

Ocusoft

Website: www.ocusoft.com

This product is a leave-on eyelid cleanser that removes oil, debris, pollen, and other contaminants from the eyelid, effectively relieving irritation. It also has anti-inflammatory properties. It is indicated for moderate to severe blepharitis, which can lead to dry eye.

Systane Lid Wipes

Systane

Website: www.systane.com

These pre-moistened eyelid cleansing wipes are designed to be used as part of a daily hygiene regimen. They remove debris and eye makeup that can cause irritation, and are hypoallergenic.

Tranquileyes

Eye Eco

Website: www.eyeeco.com

These goggles provide moisture retention and protection against dry eye by employing a deep cushion seal and removable moisture pads. Padded with comfortable memory foam, this product creates total darkness, keeps the eyelids closed, and increases humidity around the eyes.

EYE DROPS

While your doctor may prescribe an eye drop in your case, the following eye drops are available by prescription.

Product	Company	Indication/Action
Blink Gel Tears	Johnson & Johnson	Encourages longer tear retention time.
Blink Tears	Johnson & Johnson	Reduces high salt levels in the tear film.
Blink Tears Preservative-Free Drops	Johnson & Johnson	Blink Tears formulated with no preservatives.
Clear Eyes Artificial Tears	Prestige Consumer Healthcare	Preservative-free lubricant.
FreshKote	Focus Labs	Supports the integrity of all layers of the tear film.
GenTeal Tears Mild Liquid Drops	Alcon	Protects the eye against further irritation.

Product	Company	Indication/Action
GenTeal Tears Moderate Liquid Drops	Alcon	Provides fast relief from burning and irritation.
GenTeal Tears Preservative-Free Moderate Liquid Drops	Alcon	Provides fast relief and protection for those with sensitive eyes.
GenTeal Tears Severe Eye Ointment	Alcon	Provides lasting relief of dry eyes. To be used at night.
GenTeal Tears Severe Gel Lubricant Drops	Alcon	Provides lasting relief of dry eyes. To be used at night.
Oasis Preservative-Free Lubricant Eye Drops	Oasis Medical, Inc	Relieves gritty dry sensations that cause irritation.
Refresh Liquigel/ Celluvisc	Allergan	Provides extra-strength moisturizing relief plus protection for sensitive eyes.
Refresh Optive Advanced/PF	Allergan	Lubricates and hydrates the eye and protects tears from evaporation.
Refresh Optive Mega-3	Allergan	Protects tears from evaporation while nourishing the tear film damaged by dry eye. Formulated with a blend of natural oils.
Refresh Optive Repair	Allergan	Repairs the eye's dry, damaged surface.
Refresh Optive Sensitive	Allergan	Offers a unique dual-action formula that lubricates and hydrates the eye.
Refresh Tear Plus	Allergan	Mimics the soothing properties of natural tears. Formulated for sensitive eyes.
Refresh Tears	Allergan	Mimics the soothing properties of natural tears.
Retaine MGD	Ocusoft	Lipid-replenishing formula utilizes electrostatic attraction to stabilize the tear film and protect against moisture loss.

Product	Company	Indication/Action
Rhoto Dry Aid	The Mentholatum Company	Restores moisture to the tear film by working on all three layers to mimic a healthy tear.
Soothe PF	Bausch + Lomb	Restores the lipid layer and seals in moisture. Formulated for sensitive eyes.
Soothe XP	Bausch + Lomb	Restores the lipid layer, seals in moisture, and protects against further irritation.
Systane Balance	Alcon	Designed to keep the eyes feeling moist and refreshed during the day.
Systane Gel	Alcon	Offers a long-lasting formula. To be used at nighttime.
Systane Ultra	Alcon	Delivers extended protection and high-performance dry eye symptom relief that lasts.
Thera Tears Dry Eye Therapy	Akorn	Uses a unique preserving ingredient that turns into pure oxygen and water on eye contact.
Thera Tears Extra	Akorn	Offers a hypotonic and electrolyte-balanced formula to replicate healthy tears.
Thera Tears Liquid Gel	Akorn	Provides long-lasting relief and protection. For nighttime use.

$\mathscr{R}$eferences

Chapter 1

Anshel, Jeffrey. *Smart Medicine for Your Eyes*. Garden City Park, NY: Square One Publishers, 2011.

Chapter 2

Bron, AJ, De Paiva, CS, Chauhan, SK, & et al. "TFOS DEWS II Pathophysiology Report." *Ocul Surf*. 2017 Jul; 15(3): 438–510.

Khanal S, Tomlnson A, Diaper CJ. "Tear physiology of aqueous deficiency and evaporative dry eye." *Optom Vis Sci*. Nov; 86(11):1235–40.

Vehof J, Sillevis Smitt-Kamminga N, Nibourg S, et al. "Predictors of Discordance between Symptoms and Signs in Dry Eye Disease." *Ophthalmology* 2017 Mar; 124(3):280–286.

Chapter 3

Ablamowicz A, Nichols JJ, Nichols KK. "Association between serum levels of testosterone and estradiol with meibomian gland assessments in postmenopausal women." *Invest Ophthalmol Vis Sci*. 2016; 57:295–300.

Abraham, S. "Corneal complications of vernal keratoconjunctivitis." *Curr Opin Allergy Clin Immunol*. 2015 Oct. 15(5), 489–494.

Arita R, Fukuoka S, Morishige N. "Meibomina gland dysfunction and contact lens discomfort." *Eye Contact Lens* 2017; 43(1):14–9.

Arita R, Itoh K, Maeda S, et al. "Comparison of the long-term effects of various topical antiglaucoma medications on meibomian glands." *Cornea* 2012; 31:1229–34.

Ayaki M, Tsubota K, Kawashima M, et al. "Sleep Disorders are a Prevalent and Serious Comorbidity in Dry Eye." *Invest Ophthalmol Vis Sci*. 2018 Nov 1; 59(14):DES143-DES150.

Baudouin C, Messmer EM, Aragona P, et al. "Revisiting the vicious circle of dry eye disease: a focus on the pathophysiology of Meibomian gland dysfunction." *Br j Ophthalmol*. 2016; 100(3):300–6.

Bierdeman M, Torres AM, Caballero AR, Tang A, O'Callaghan RJ. (2017). "Reactions with antisera and pathological effects of staphylococcus aureus gamma-toxin in the cornea." *Curr Eye Res*. 2017 Mar 27:1–8(10.1080/02713683.2017.1279636.)

Blackie CA, Solomon JD, Scaffidi RC, et al. "The relationship between dry eye symptoms and lipid layer thickness." *Cornea* 2009 Aug; 28(7):789–94.

Brent GA. "Graves' disease." *N Engl J Med*. 2008; 358:2544–54.

Calonge, Margarita MD, PhD; Pinto-Fraga, Jose OD, MSc; González-García, María J. OD, PhD; et al. "Effects of the External Environment on Dry Eye Disease." *International Ophthalmology Clinics* April 2017. Volume 57, Issue 2: p 23–40.

Chen L, Pi L, Fang J, et al. "High incidence of dry eye in young children with allergic conjunctivitis in Southwest China." *Acta Ophthalmol*. 2016 Dec; 94(8):e727-e730.

Choi YJ, Park SY, Jun I, et al. "Perioperative Ocular Parameters Associated With Persistent Dry Eye Symptoms After Cataract Surgery." *Cornea* 2018 Jun; 37(6):734–739.

Erdem U, Ozdegirmenci O, Sobaci E, et al. "Dry eye in post-menopausal women using hormone replacement therapy." *Maturitas* 2007 Mar 20; 56(3):257–62.

Ficker L, Seal D, Wright P. "Staphylococcal infection and the limbus: Study of the cell-mediated immune response." *Eye* 1989; 3: 190–193.

Flores-Páez LA., Zenteno JC, Alcántar-Curiel MD, Vargas-Mendoza CF, Rodríguez-Martínez, S, Cancino-Diaz, ME, et al. "Molecular and phenotypic characterization of staphylococcus epidermidis isolates from healthy conjunctiva and a comparative analysis with isolates from ocular infection." *PLoS One* (eCollection 2015); 10(8): 07/31/2017.

Gaikwad SL, Gaikwad R, Akil M, Ramsay HM. "Contact allergy masquerading as seronegative Sjögren's syndrome." *Oral Surg Oral Med Oral Pathol Oral Radiol*. 2013 Nov; 116(5):e375–8.

Gao Y, Di Pascuale M, Li W, et al. "High prevalence of ocular Demodex in lashes with cylindrical dandruffs." *Invest Ophthalmol Vis Sci*. 2005; 46:3089–3094.

Ghanem VC, Mehra N, Wong S, Mannis MJ. "The prevalence of ocular signs in acne rosacea: comparing patients from ophthalmology and dermatology clinics." *Cornea* 2003; 22(3):230–3.

Goebbels M. "Tear secretion and tear film function in insulin dependent diabetics." *Br J Ophthalmol* 2000; 84(1):19–21.

Golebiowski B, Badarudin N, Eden J, et al. "Does endogenous serum estrogen play a role in meibomian gland dysfunction in postmenopausal women with dry eye?" *Br J Ophthalmol*. 2016: 1–6.

Grus FH, Sabuncuo P, Dick HB, et al. "Changes in the tear proteins of diabetic patients." *BMC Ophthalmol*. 2002; 2(1):4.

Gunay M, Celik G, Yidiz E, et al. "Ocular surface characteristics in diabetic children." *Curr Eye Res*. 2016 Dec; 41(12):1526–31.

Gurdal C, Sarac O, Genc I, et al. "Ocular surface and dry eye in Grave's disease." *Curr Eye Res*. 2011; 36(1):8–13.

Hirota M, Uozato H, Kawamorita T, et al. "Effect of Incomplete Blinking on Tear Film Stability." *Optom Vis Sci*. 2013; 90:650–657.

Hussein, N., & Schwab, I. R. (2013). Chapter 22: blepharitis and inflammation of the eyelids. In W. Tasman, & E. A. Jaeger (Eds.), *Duane's Ophthalmology* (12th Edition ed., pp. Volume 4). 530 Walnut Street, Philadelphia, PA 19106 USA: Lippincott Williams & Wilkins.

Jaanus SD, Bartlett JD, Hlett, JA. *Ocular Effects of Systemic Drugs*. Bartlett JD & Jaanus SD (eds.). Clinical Ocular Pharmacology 3rd ed. Boston: Butterworth-Heinemann; 1995:957–1006.

Jain, S. "Dry eyes in diabetes." *Diabetes Care* 1998:21 (8):1375; discussion 1375–6.

Jayamanne DG, Dayan M, Jenkins D, & et al. "The role of staphylococcal super-antigens in the pathogenesis of marginal keratitis." *Eye* 1997; 11; 618–621.

Jun Hyung Moon, Kyoung Woo Kim, Nam Ju Moon. "Smartphone use is a risk factor for pediatric dry eye disease according to region and age: a case control study." *BMC Ophthalmology* 2016; 16:188.

Kawashima M1, Uchino M2, Yokoi N3, et al. "The association of sleep quality with dry eye disease: the Osaka study." *Clin Ophthalmol*. 2016 Jun 1; 10:1015–21.

Kawashima M, Uchino M, Yokoi N, et al. "The association of sleep quality with dry eye disease: the Osaka study." *Clin Ophthalmol*. 2016 Jun 1; 10:1015–21.

Kheirkhah, A., Casas, V., Li, W., Raju, V. K., & Tseng, S. C. (2007 May). Corneal manifestations of ocular demodex infestation. *Am J Ophthalmol*, 143(5), 743–749.

Kılıç Müftüoglu, I., & Aydın Akova, Y. "Clinical findings, follow-up and treatment results in patients with ocular rosacea." *Turkish Journal of Ophthalmology* 2016; 46(1): 1–6.

Kivanc SA, Kivanc M, Bayramlar H. "Microbiology of corneal wounds after cataract surgery: biofilm formation and antibiotic resistance pattern." *J Wound Care* 2016; 25(1):12, 14–19.

Kohli P, Arya SK, Raj A, et al. "Changes in ocular surface status after phacoemulsification in patients with senile cataract." *Int Ophthalmol.* 2018 Jun 20.

Lee SH, Oh DH, Jung JY, et al. "Comparative ocular microbial communities in humans with and without blepharitis." *Invest Ophthalmol Vis Sci.* 2012 Aug 15; 53(9): 5585–5593.

Leung EW, Medeiros FA, Weinreb RN. "Prevalence of ocular surface disease in glaucoma patients." *Journal of Glaucoma* 2008; 17: 350–5.

Lilleby V, Gran JT. "Systemic rheumatoid arthritis." *Tidsskr Nor Laegeforen* 1997 Nov 30; 117(29): 4223–5.

Liu S, Hatton MP, Khandelwal P, Sullivan DA. "Culture, immortalization, and characterization of human meibomian gland epithelial cells." *Invest Ophthalmol Vis Sci* 2010; 51(8): 3993–4005.

López-Valverde G, Garcia-Martin E, Larrosa-Povés JM, Polo-Llorens V, Pablo-Júlvez LE. "Therapeutical management for ocular rosacea." *Case Rep Ophthalmol.* 2016 May; 7(1): 237–242.

Lubis RR, Gultom MTH. "The Correlation between Daily Lens Wear Duration and Dry Eye Syndrome." Open Access *Maced J Med Sci.* 2018 May 18; 6(5): 829–834.

Maier P, Lapp T, Reinhard T. "Ocular involvement in atopic dermatitis: Clinical aspects and therapy." *Ophthalmologe.* 2017 Jun; 114(6):514–524.

Mastrota KM. "Impact of floppy eyelid syndrome in ocular surface and dry eye disease." *Optom Vis Sci.* 2008 Sep; 85(9): 814–6.

Mathers WD, Stovall D, Land JA, et al. "Menopause and tear function: the influence of prolactin and sex hormones on human tear production." *Cornea* 1998 Jul; 17(4): 353–8.

McCulley J. "Systemic and autoimmune disease that lead to dry eye." www.ophthalmologymanagement.co/articleviewer.aspx?articleID=105864. Accessed Aug. 30, 2018.

Medscape. "Ophthalmologic Manifestations of Sjögren's Syndrome." http://emedicine.medscape.com/article/1192919overview. Accessed Sept. 17, 2018.

Moon JF, Kim KW, Moon NJ. "Smartphone use is a risk factor for pediatric dry eye disease according to region and age: a case control study." *BMC Ophthalmol.* 2016 Oct. 28; 167(1): 188.

Muchnick BG. "Identify the ocular side effects of systemic medications." *Rev Optom.* 2008 Jan; 145(1):60–73.

Nichols KK, Nichols JJ, Mitchell GL. "The lack of association between signs and symptoms in patients with dry eye disease." *Cornea* 2004; 23(8):762–70.

Nikole L. Himebaugh, OD, Debra R. Renner, OD, Carolyn G. Begley, OD, MS. "Blink Rate, Fullness of Blink, and Tear Film Break-Up with Four Different Visual Tasks." Indiana University School of Optometry.

Ozdemir, M. Buyukbese, MA Centinkaya, A, et al. "Risk factors for ocular surface disorders in patients with diabetes mellitus." *Diabetes Res Clin Pract* 2003; 59(3): 195–9.

Ra S, Ayaki M1, Yuki K. "Dry eye, sleep quality, and mood status in glaucoma patients receiving prostaglandin monotherapy were comparable with those in non-glaucoma subjects." *PLoS One* 2017 Nov 27; 12(11):e0188534.

Rehman H. "Sjögren's syndrome." *Yonsei Med J* 2003 Dec 20; 44(4); 947–54.

Rossi GC, Pasinetti GM, Scudeller L, Raimondi M, Lanteri S, Bianchi PE. "Risk factors to develop ocular surface disease in treated glaucoma or ocular hypertension patients." *European Journal of Ophthalmology* 2013; 23: 296–302.

Rynerson JM, Perry HD. "DEBS- a unification theory for dry eye and blepharitis." *Clin Ophthalmol.* 2016;10: 2455–67.

Sanming Li, Ke Ning, Jing Zhou, et al. "Sleep deprivation disrupts the lacrimal system and induces dry eye disease." *Experimental & Molecular Medicine* 2018 Volume 50; e451.

Schaumberg DA, Buring JE, Sullivan DA, et al. "Hormone replacement therapy and dry eye syndrome." *JAMA* 2001 Nov 7; 286(17): 2114–9.

Schaumberg DA, Nichols JJ, Papas EB, et al. "The international workshop on meibomian gland dysfunction: report of the subcommittee on the epidemiology of, and associated risk factors for, MGD." *Invest Ophthalmol Vis Sci.* 2011; 52(4): 1994–2005.

Schaumberg DA, Sullivan DA, Buring JE, et al. "Prevalence of dry eye syndrome among US women." *Am J Ophthalmol* 2003; 136(2): 318–26.

Seal D, Ficker L, Ramakrishnan M, et al." Role of staphylococcal toxin production in blepharitis." *Ophthalmology* 1990; 97(12), 1684–1688.

Shao D, Zhu X, Sun W, et al. "Effects of femtosecond laser-assisted cataract surgery on dry eye." *Exp Ther Med.* 2018 Dec; 16(6): 5073–5078.

Sivaraj RR, Durrani OM, Denniston AK, et al. "Ocular manifestations of systemic lupus erythematosus." *Rheumatology* 2007 Dec; 46(12): 1757–62.

Song P, Xia W, Wang M, et al. "Variations of dry eye disease prevalence by age, sex and geographic characteristics in China: a systematic review and meta-analysis." *J Glob Health* 2018 Dec; 8(2): 020503.

Sullivan DA, Jensen RV, Suzuki T, Richards SM. "Do sex steroids exert sex-specific and/or opposite effects on gene expression in lacrimal and meibomian glands?" *Mol Vis.* 2009; 15: 1553–72.

Suzuki T. "Inflamed Obstructive Meibomian Gland Dysfunction Causes Ocular Surface Inflammation." *Invest Ophthalmol Vis Sci.* 2018 Nov 1;59(14): DES94-DES101.

Suzuki T, Mitsuishi Y, Sano Y, Yokoi N, Kinoshita S. "Phlyctenular keratitis associated with meibomitis in young patients." *American Journal of Ophthalmology* 2005; 140(1): 77.e1–77.e7.

Taner P, Akarsu C, Atasoy P, et al. "The effects of hormone replacement therapy on ocular surface and tear function tests in postmenopausal women." *Ophthalmologica* 2004 Jul-Aug; 218(4): 257–9.

Tetz MR, Klein U, V. H. "Staphylococcus-associated blepharokeratoconjunctivitis. Clinical findings, pathogenesis and therapy." *Ophthalmologe* 1997; 94(3): 186–190.

Thody AJ, Shuster S. "Control and function of sebaceous glands." *Physiol Rev.* 1989; 69(2): 383–416.

Thygeson, P. (1969). "Complications of staphylococcic blepharitis." doi:http://dx.doi.org/10.1016/0002–9394(69)90711–9.

Truong S, Cole N, Stapleton F, Golebiowski B. "Sex hormones and the dry eye." *Clin Exp Optom.* 2014; 97: 324–336.

Ueta M, Sotozono C, Takahashi J, Kojima K, Ueta M. "Examination of staphylococcus aureus on the ocular surface of patients with catarrhal ulcers." *Cornea* 2009, Aug; 28(7): 780–782.

Uncu G, Avci R, Uncu Y, et al. "The effects of different hormone replacement therapy regimens on tear function, intraocular pressure and lens opacity." *Gynecol Endocrinol* 2006 Sep; 22(9): 501–5.

Uzunosmanoglu E, Mocan MC, Kocabeyoglu S, Karakaya J, Irkec M. "Meibomian Gland Dysfunction in Patients Receiving Long-Term Glaucoma Medications." *Cornea* 2016; 35: 1112–6.

Vishnubhatla S, Borchman D, Foulks GN. "Contact lenses and the rate of evaporation measured in vitro; the influence of wear, squalene and wax." *Cont Lens Anterior Eye* 2012; 35(6): 277–81.

Wolffsohn JS, Arita R, Chalmers R, et al. "TFOS DEWS II Diagnostic Methodology report." *Ocul Surf.* 2017 Jul; 15(3): 539–74.

Wong, Victoria M MedSc, Lai, Timothy MD, Chi, Stanley, Lam, Dennis MD, Ophth. "Pediatric ocular surface infections: A 5-year review of demographics, clinical features, risk factors, microbiological results, and treatment." *Cornea* 2011; 30(9): 995–1002.

Zlatanovi G, Velelinovi D, Cki S, et al. "Ocular manifestation of rheumatoid arthritis-different forms and frequency." *Bosn J Basic Med Sci* Nov; 10(4): 323–7.

Chapter 5

Azari AA, Rapuano CJ. "Autologous serum eye drops for the treatment of ocular surface disease." *Eye Contact Lens* 2015 May; 41(3): 133–140.

Bavinger JC, DeLoss K, Mian SI. "Scleral lens use in dry eye syndrome." *Curr Opin Ophthalmol.* 2015; 26: 319–24.

Chahal HS, Estrada M, Sindt CW, et al. "Scleral Contact Lenses in an Academic Oculoplastics Clinic: Epidemiology and Emerging Considerations." *Ophthalmic Plast Reconstr Surg.* 2018 May/Jun; 34(3): 231–236.

Cheng AM, Zhao D, Chen R, Yin, HY, Tighe S, Sheha H, et al. "Accelerated restoration of ocular surface health in dry eye disease by self-retained cryopreserved amniotic membrane." *Ocul Surf.* 216 Jan; 14(1): 56–63.

Cho YK, Huang W, Kim GY, Lim, BS. "Comparison of autologous serum eye drops with different diluents." *Curr Eye Res* 2013, Jan; 38(1): 9–17.

Doll, Tracy. "Cryopreserved Amniotic Membrane, Autologous Serum Eye Drops, and Tea-Tree Oil Lid Scrubs in combination for the treatment of Keratoconjunctivitis in a Staphylococcus Hyperacnsitive Teenager." Pacific University College of Optometry Vol 1 No 1 (2018): *Journal of Dry Eye Disease.*

Fischer KR, Opitz A, Böeck M, Geerling G. "Stability of serum eye drops after storage of 6 months." *Cornea* 2012 Nov; 31(11): 1313–1318.

Jeng BH, Dupps WJJ. "Autologous serum 50% eyedrops in the treatment of persistent corneal epithelial defects." *Cornea* 2009 Dec; 28(10): 1104 1108.

Kojima T, Higuchi A, Goto E, Matsumoto Y, Dogru M, Tsubota K. "Autologous serum eye drops for the treatment of dry eye diseases." *Cornea* 2008 Sep; 27(Suppl 1): S25-S30.

Semeraro F, Forbice E, Braga O, Bova A, Di Salvatore A, Azzolini C. "Evaluation of the efficacy of 50% autologous serum eye drops in different ocular surface pathologies." *BioMed Research International* 826970, 2017 Jul 31.

Sheha H, Liang L, Li J, Tseng SC. "Sutureless amniotic membrane transplantation for severe bacterial keratitis." *Cornea* 2009 Dec; 28(10): 1118–1123.

Tabatabaei SA, Soleimani M, Behrouz MJ, Torkashvand A, Anvari P, Yaseri M. "A randomized clinical trial to evaluate the usefulness of amniotic membrane transplantation in bacterial keratitis healing." *Ocul Surf.* 2017 Apr; 15(2): 218–226.

Toyos R, McGill W, Briscoe D, "Intense pulsed light treatment for dry eye disease due to meibomian gland dysfunction; a 3-year retrospective study." *Photomedicine and Laser Surgery* 2015 Jan; 33(1): 41–46. doi:10.1089/pho.2014.3819. ISSN 1557-8550. PMC 4298157?Freely accessible.

Vegunta S, Patel, Dharmendra S, Joanne F. "Combination Therapy of Intense

Pulsed Light Therapy and Meibomian Gland Expression (IPL/MGX) Can Improve Dry Eye Symptoms and Meibomian Gland Function in Patients with Refractory Dry Eye: A Retrospective Analysis." *Cornea* 2016 Mar; 35(3): 318–322.

Vora GK, Gupta, PK. "Intense pulsed light therapy for the treatment of evaporative dry eye disease." *Current Opinion in Ophthalmology* 2015 July; 26(4): 314–318.

Yang J, Yang F, Peng C, et al. "Surgical treatment of 32 cases of long-term atopic keratoconjunctivitis using the amniotic membrane." *Eye* 2013; 27(11): 1254–1262.

Chapter 6

Adam O, Wolfram G, Zollner N. "Effect of alpha-linolenic acid in the human diet on linoleum acid metabolism and prostaglandin biosynthesis." *J Lipid Res.* 1986; 27(4): 421–6.

Burstein NL. "The effects of topical drugs and preservatives on the tears and corneal epithelium in dry eye." *Trans Ophthalmol Soc U K.* 1985; 104(Pt 4): 402–409.

Calder PC. "n-3 polyunsaturated fatty acids, inflammation and inflammatory diseases." *Am J Clin Nutr.* 2006; 83(6 suppl): 1505S-19S.

Carnahan MC, Goldstein DA. "Ocular complications of topical, peri-ocular, and systemic corticosteroids." *Current Opinion in Ophthalmology* 2000; 11(6): 478–483.

Cox SD, Mann CM, Markham JL, Bell HC, Gustafson JE, Warmington JR, et al. "The mode of antimicrobial action of the essential oil of melaleuca alternifolia (tea tree oil)." *J Appl Microbiol.* 2000 Jan; 88(1): 170–175.

Daniel BS, Orchard D. "Ocular side-effects of topical corticosteroids: What a dermatologist needs to know." *Australas J Dermatol* 20115 Aug; 56(3): 164–169.

Epstein SP, Gadaria-Rathod N, Wei Y, et al. "HLA-DR expression as a biomarker of inflammation for multicenter clinical trials of ocular surface disease." *Exp Eye Res.* 2013;111: 95–104.

Funk CD. "Prostaglandins and leukotrienes: advances in eicosanoid biology." *Science* 2001; 294(5548): 1871–5.

Hammer KA, Carson CF, Riley TV. "Effects of melaleuca alternifolia (tea tree) essential oil and the major monoterpene component terpinen-4-ol on the development of single- and multistep antibiotic resistance and antimicrobial susceptibility." *Antimicrobial Agents and Chemotherapy* 2012; 56(2): 909–915.

Harauma A, Saigon J, Watanabe Y, et al. "Potential for daily supplementation of n-3 fatty acids to reverse symptoms of dry eye in mice." *Prostaglandins Leuko Essential Fatty Acids* 2014; 90(6): 207–13.

Healy DA, Wallace FA, Miles EA, et al. "Effect of low to moderate amounts of dietary fish oil on neutrophil lipid composition and function." *Lipids* 2000; 35(7): 763–8.

Hom MM, Asbell P, Barry B. "Omegas and dry eye: more knowledge, more questions." *Optom Vis Sci.* 2015; 92(9): 948–56.

Homeyer D, Sanchez CJ, Mende K, et al. "In vitro activity of melaleuca alternifolia (tea tree) oil on filamentous fungi and toxicity to human cells." *Medical Mycology* 2015 Apr; 53(3): 285–294.

Hong S, Gronert K, Devchand PR, et al. "Novel docosatrienes and 17S-resolvins generated from docosahexaenoic acids in murine brain, human blood, and glial cells. Autacoids in anti-inflammation." *J Biol Chem.* 2003; 278(17): 14677–87.

Jackson MA, Burrell K, Gaddie I, Richardson SD. "Efficacy of a new prescription omega only medical food supplement in alleviating signs and symptoms of dry eye, with or without concomitant cyclosporine A." *Clin Ophthalmol.* 2011; 5: 1201–6.

Kangari II, Eftekhari MII, Sardari S, et al. "Short-term consumption of oral omega-3 and dry eye syndrome." *Ophthalmology* 2013; 120(11): 2191–6.

Kawakita T, Kawabata F, Tsui T, et al. "Effects of dietary supplementation with fish oil on dry eye syndrome subjects: randomized controlled trial." *Biomed Res.* 2013; 34(5): 215–20.

Koo H, Kim TH, Kim KW, Wee SW, Chun YS, Kim JC. "Ocular surface discomfort and demodex: Effect of tea tree oil eyelid scrub in demodex Blepharitis." *Journal of Korean Medical Science* 2012; 27(12): 1574–1579.

Kwok A, Lam D, Ng J, et al. "Ocular-hypertensive response to topical steroids in children." *Ophthalmology* 1997; 104(12), 2112–2116.

Li N, Ho J, Schwartz CE, Gjorstrup P, Bazan HE. "Resolvin F1 improves tear production and decreases inflammation in a dry eye mouse model." *J Ocul Pharmacol Ther.* 2010; 26(5): 431–9.

Liu A, Ji J. "Omega-3 essential fatty acid therapy for dry eye syndrome: a meta-analysis of randomized controlled studies." *Med Sci Monit.* 2014; 20(1): 1583–9.

Massingale ML, Li X, Vallabhajosyula M, et al. "Analysis of inflammatory cytokines in the tears of dry eye patients." *Cornea* 2009; 28(9): 1023–7.

Oum BS, Kim NM, Lee JS, et al. "Effects of fluoroquinolone eye solutions without preservatives on human corneal epithelial cells in vitro." *Ophthalmic Res.* 2014; 51: 216–223.

Renfro L, Snow JS. "Ocular effects of topical and systemic steroids." *Dermatol Clin.* 1992 Jul; 10(3): 505–512.

Simopoulos, AP. "Essential fatty acids in health and chronic disease." *Am J Clin Nutr.* 1999; 70(suppl): 560S-9S.

Surette ME. "The science behind dietary omega 3 fatty acids." *Can Med Assoc J.* 2008; 178(2): 177–80.

Thomsen NA, Hammer KA, Riley TV, Van Belkum A, Carson CF. "Effect of habituation to tea tree (melaleuca alternifolia) oil on the subsequent susceptibility of staphylococcus spp. to antimicrobials, triclosan, tea tree oil, terpinen-4-ol and carvacrol." *Int J Antimicrob Agents* 2013 Apr. 4(41): 343–351.

Walter SD, Gronert K, McClellan AL, et al. "Omega 3 tear film lipids correlate with clinical measures of dry eye." *Invest Ophthalmol Vis Sci.* 2016; 57(6): 2472–8.

Wei Y, Gadaria-Rathod N, Epstein S, et al. "Tear cytokine profile as a noninvasive biomarker of inflammation for ocular surface diseases: standard operating procedures." *Invest Ophthalmol Vis Sci.* 2013; 54(13): 8327–36.

Zhang S, Zhu YT, Chen SY, et al. "Constitutive expression of pentraxin 3 (PTX3) protein by human amniotic membrane cells leads to formation of the heavy chain (HC)-hyaluronan (HA)-PTX3 complex." *J Biol Chem.* 2014; 289: 13531–13542.

Zhao Y, Joshi-Barve S, Barve S, et al. "Eicosapentaenoic acid prevents LPS-induced TNF-alpha expression by preventing NF-kappaB activation." *J Am Coll Nutr.* 2004; 23(1): 71–8.

Zhu W, Wu Y, Li G, et al. "Efficacy of polyunsaturated fatty acids for dry eye syndrome: a meta-analysis of randomized controlled trials." *Nutr Rev.* 2014; 72(10): 662–71.

Chapter 7

Francois CA, Connor SL, Bolewicz LC, et al. "Supplementing lactating women with flaxseed oil does not increase docosahexaenoic acid in their milk." *Am J Clin Nutr.* 2003 Jan; 77(1): 226–33.

Sheppard JD Jr, Singh R, McClellan, et al. "Long-term Supplementation with n-6 and n-3 PUFAs Improves Moderate-to-Severe Keratoconjunctivitis Sicca: A Randomized Double-Blind Clinical Trial." *Cornea* 2013 Oct; Volume 32, Issue 10: p 1297–1304.

Vasquez A. "Reducing pain and inflammation naturally. Part II: new insights into fatty acid supplementation and its effect on eicosanoid production and genetic expression." *Nutritional Perspectives J Counc Nutr Am Chiro Assoc.* 2005; 28(1): 5–16.

$\mathcal{I}$ndex

OTHER SQUAREONE TITLES OF INTEREST

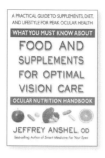

What You Must Know About Food and Supplements for Optimal Vision Care

Jeffrey Anshel, OD

Over the last twenty years, more and more studies have demonstrated that certain foods and natural supplements can play a supportive role in the treatment of a number of eye problems. This book is a concise, easy-to-read guide to these powerful substances.

$16.95 US • 176 pages • 6 x 9-inch paperback • ISBN 978-0-7570-0410-0

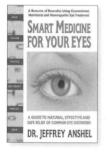

What You Must Know About Age-Related Macular Degeneration

Jeffrey Anshel, OD , and Laura Stevens, M.Sci

Age-related macular degeneration (AMD) is the most commonly diagnosed eye disorder in people over fifty. Best-selling authors Dr. Jeffrey Anshel and Laura Stevens have written this comprehensive guide to preventing, treating, or even reversing this condition through nutritional supplements, the Anti-AMD Diet, and simple lifestyle changes.

$17.95 US • 224 pages • 6 x 9-inch paperback • ISBN 978-0-7570-0449-0

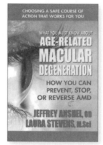

Smart Medicine for Your Eyes

Jeffrey Anshel, OD

This book is an A-to-Z guide to eye disorders and their conventional and alternative treatments. Divided into three parts, this easy-to-understand book begins with an overview of eye function in Part One and introduce methods of treatment from acupuncture to nutrition. Part Two is a comprehensive directory of eye disorders and their therapy options, and Part Three guides you in using the recommended procedures.

$19.95 US • 424 pages • 7.5 x 9-inch paperback • ISBN 978-0-7570-0301-1

High Performance Vision

Donald S. Teig, OD

Beyond physical superiority and mental stamina, most of the world's best athletes possess another advantage: good vision. Maximizing your vision can mean the difference between being a good player and a great one. If you've been looking for a natural way to enhance your eyesight and take your game to the next level, *High Performance Vision* will show you how.

$17.95 US • 176 pages • 6 x 9-inch paperback • ISBN 978-0-7570-0399-8

For more information about our books,
visit our website at www.squareonepublishers.com